This book's home
is at Shirley Ann
58750 Peb...
Vermonia, Oregon #97064
(429-5813)

P9-BIU-924

Mushrooms:
Wild and Edible

Shirley Ely's
4/295313

VINCENT MARTEKA

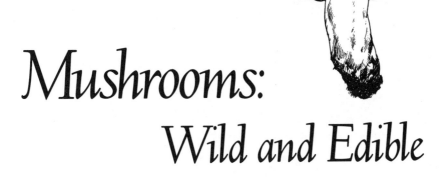

Mushrooms:
Wild and Edible

A Seasonal Guide to the
Most Easily Recognized Mushrooms

W·W·NORTON & COMPANY

NEW YORK   LONDON

The recipe for chanterelles on toast is from *The Wild Gourmet*, by Babette Brackett and Maryann Lash. Copyright © 1975 by David R. Godine. Reprinted by permission of David R. Godine, Publisher, Inc.

Copyright © 1980 by Vincent Marteka

Published simultaneously in Canada by George J. McLeod Limited, Toronto. Printed in the United States of America.
All Rights Reserved
First Edition

Illustration credits appear on p. 275.

BOOK DESIGN BY EARL TIDWELL

Library of Congress Cataloging in Publication Data

Marteka, Vincent J
    Mushrooms, wild and edible.

    Bibliography: p.
    Includes index.
    1. Mushrooms, Edible—United States—Identification. 2. Cookery (Mushrooms) I. Title.
QK617.M413 1980   641.3'58   80–13910
ISBN 0–393–01356–1

1 2 3 4 5 6 7 8 9 0

To My Mother and Father

who, like many other Americans
of Polish ancestry, transplanted
their love of edible mushrooms
to their son in a new land.

Contents

List of Illustrations

SEASONAL DRAWINGS

COLOR PLATES (*following page 144*)

Introduction

For many years I have felt the need for a book on mushrooms that would introduce a beginner simply and safely to the fascinating world of edible fungi. Such a book, I felt, should be limited to the most easily identified edible species that are widespread in the United States; should have outstanding color photos and other key illustrations that would make it easy to identify a mushroom; should be arranged seasonally, so that a mushroomer would know exactly what mushroom to look for in what season and not waste time looking for some other mushroom that would appear later; should be interesting and pleasurable reading, going beyond the usual brief description of mushrooms, so that when a person finished reading about the mushroom, he or she could honestly say "I know that mushroom"; and, finally, the book should introduce the reader to the pleasurable world of edible mushrooms by providing a selection of tantalizing recipes.

I believe that this book meets these various needs of the beginner. My hope is that it will prove valuable to the experienced mushroom collector as well, to the person who wishes to expand his knowledge of mushrooms, whether it be in cultivating mushrooms at home or exploring the contributions that mushrooms have made to the various cuisines of the world.

Happy mushroom hunting to all!

VINCENT MARTEKA

October, 1979

Acknowledgments

My sincere thanks go to Dr. Clark T. Rogerson, senior curator of the New York Botanical Garden and past president of the Mycological Society of America, for reading Part I and Part II of the book for technical accuracy; to Margaret Lewis of the Boston Mycological Club for reading the sections in Part III on preserving and preparing wild mushrooms; and to Dr. Donald Simons, du Pont chemist, toxicology expert, and chairman of the North American Mycological Association's committee on mushroom toxicology, for reading the chapter on poisonous mushrooms. Special recognition should go to Neal MacDonald, the artist who graced this book with illustrations that combine meticulous technical accuracy with fine artistry. And finally my deepest thanks to my patient wife Janet, for her culinary contributions and for typing the entire book manuscript.

Part I

Entering the World of Mushrooms

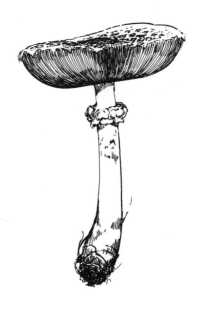

What Is a Mushroom?

Mushrooms belong to that large group of simple plants known as fungi. An estimated 300,000 species of fungi exist in the world. These widely distributed organisms are the most common non-flowering plants on earth. Fungi grow in the soil, on wood, in water, on plants, and even on humans. They range in size from the microscopic molds that cover old bread to the large bracket mushrooms that form shelves on wood 3 feet or more in width. Some fungi are harmful to humans, whole others are very beneficial. The wonder drug penicillin is obtained from the *Penicillium* fungus, and yeast fungi have been used for centuries to ferment food or drink. Other fungi such as rust may extensively damage wheat crops, while molds may decay leather.

Unlike the typical green plants with which you are familiar, fungi have no roots, flowers, seeds, or leaves. They do not contain chlorophyll. The chlorophyll in green plants taps the energy of sunlight to make plant food from the carbon dioxide in the air and from water and minerals in the soil. Without chlorophyll, fungi have to rely on food material produced by other plants and animals. This material may, for example, be actual growing plants or the remains of organisms such as fallen leaves in the soil.

The study of fungi is known as *mycology*, from the Greek

word *mykes,* "fungus." Although microscopic fungi such as molds and yeasts are fascinating, it is the larger fungi—the mushrooms—that interest most people.

The word *mushroom* is believed to have originated from the French word *mousseron,* which, in turn, was derived from the word *mousse* or moss. The popular usage of the word *mushroom* varies considerably. Many people call all large fungi with a cap and a stem a mushroom. Others limit the term to any edible mushroom, while designating all poisonous fungi as toadstools. To confuse the situation still further, the words *mushroom* and *toadstool* are used interchangeably by some people when referring to all mushrooms.

Mycologists, scientists who study fungi, may use the term *mushroom* to refer to any fungus that has bladelike gills underneath the cap. These gills radiate from the mushroom stem like spokes on a wheel. This group of gilled mushrooms is known as Agaricales, or agarics.

In more recent years, the popular usage of the term *mushroom* among amateur and professional mycologists has been considerably broadened to include any large fleshy fungi. Diverse fungi such as the puffballs, the spongelike morels, and the boletes with the underside studded with tiny pinholes now come under the mushroom umbrella. This broader usage is the one followed in this book. The term *toadstool* has been banished to the nether regions of witch's cauldrons, Shakespearean tales, and other fantasies.

How Mushrooms Are Produced

Surprisingly, what we call a mushroom is really only the fruiting part of a plant that is visible above the ground or wood on which the mushroom grows. Most of the mushroom plant, a network of tiny rootlike threads, is hidden underground or under wood. The sole purpose of the fruiting mushroom (Figure 1) is to ensure the spread of another generation of mushrooms by the releas-

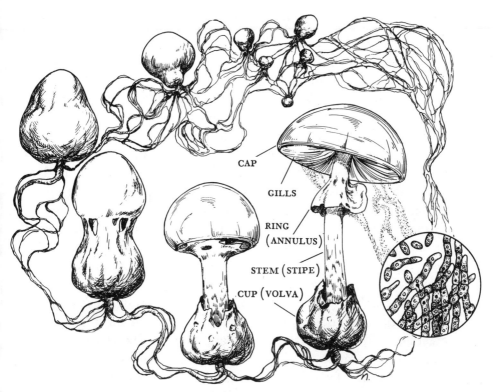

FIGURE 1. *The life cycle of a gilled mushroom (an amanita), including the main parts of a mature mushroom. Counterclockwise from lower right, the development of mycelia from spores (circle insert). Buttons develop on the mycelia, and eventually the cap and stipe emerge, forming the mature fruiting body.*

ing of tiny particles known as spores. These spores often fill the air in tremendous numbers.

In a gilled mushroom such as the amanita illustrated in Figure 1, the spores are produced on the gills. Although you cannot see the connection with the naked eye, the spores—before they are released—are attached to microscopic club-shaped cells called *basidia.* The white spores hang like Christmas tree ornaments from the basidia.

The spores are so small that 10,000 can fit into an area about the size of a small pea. The white spores of the amanita can be seen more clearly if the cap is placed on a piece of black paper after the stem has been cut off. A short time later, a white print showing the outline of the gills will show up on the paper. The print is actually made up of tiny piles containing millions of spores that rained onto the paper from the gills beneath the cap.

Normally, when the humidity of the air changes, tiny mechanisms in the basidia are triggered, causing the spores to be released. Once released, the spores are blown about by wind currents. Like a scene from a slow-motion film, the spores tumble and fall through the air. The journey is so slow that an average-sized spore takes more than ten minutes to fall 1 foot. Scientists have calculated that although about 99.9 percent of the spores descend to the ground within 100 feet of the liberating mushroom, the remaining spores may be carried long distances. Fungus spores have been detected from airplanes high in the atmosphere and over the ocean far from land.

The combined output of spores from millions of mushrooms and other fungi is staggering. Spores are in the air that you breathe, on the food that you eat, and even on the clothes that you wear. A meadow mushroom with a cap 3 inches in diameter will release 1.8 billion spores, according to calculations made earlier in this century by A. H. R. Buller, a Canadian mycologist. Not to be outdone, a Czech scientist, Albert Pilat, figured that an 8-pound puffball brought into the Prague Museum produced 1.5 trillion spores. If these tiny spores were placed side by side, they would circle the earth fifteen times.

Only a very small percentage of these spores germinate. A spore must alight in an area where conditions are ideal for its growth. If a spore of a meadow mushroom, a fungus that lives in open grassy areas, lands on a leaf or stump in a woodland, it will not germinate. However, if a spore alights in a field with a plentiful supply of food and water, it will begin to grow. A bump first appears on the spore. This bump elongates into a thread that spreads through the soil and branches further into still more threads. This small network, which resembles a fine mesh, is known as a *mycelium* (*mycelia*, plural). When the mycelium meets another mycelium, they merge and clamp together into one network. This secondary mycelium is usually the source of the fruiting mushrooms.

Periodically, when conditions are right (for example after a soaking rain), tiny bumps or knobs will appear on this secondary mycelium. These knobs will expand as they absorb water and other material. Finally, the knobs will thrust their way to the surface and emerge as the familiar fruiting body or mushroom.

A mycelium obtains food when chemical enzymes from the growing tips are released into the nearby soil. These enzymes break down food such as decayed grass or manure into material that can be absorbed by the threads. Part of this food is used to expand the mycelial network; another part will be used to produce the mushroom fruit.

The rate of growth of the mycelium depends on the amount of food available. In laboratory experiments, a speck of mycelium in a dish containing food nutrients will constantly form new branches about every half hour. Each strand of each branch may grow about 1/100ths of an inch an hour, so that in only a day or two a dish may be covered with fungus mycelia. In nature, such ideal conditions are not necessarily always present. The mycelium simply travels to the source of food. If a food supply is uniformly spread throughout the soil, an interesting circular pattern, called a fairy ring, is formed when the mycelium fruits. These circles or rings of mushrooms, according to legend, marked the path of dancing fairies.

Each year, mushrooms appear at the leading edge of this expanding circle of mycelium. If the food supply is sufficient, the circle of mycelium may expand for hundreds of years. In undisturbed prairie grasslands in Kansas, biologists have found fairy rings of meadow mushrooms and puffballs that were more than 600 feet in diameter. If the mycelium grew at a rate of about 18 inches a year, some of the rings in Kansas were formed at about the same time that Columbus landed in America, nearly 500 years ago. Large fairy rings several centuries old have also been found in England near Stonehenge. They form a perfect natural counterpoint to the circular assemblage of rocks placed by humans about 3,500 years ago to record the changing seasons through astronomical observations.

Conditions such as temperature and moisture have to be just

right before a mycelium will bear fruit. Some mushrooms will only fruit in the cold temperatures of fall, after the first frosts have finished the vegetable garden for the year and the wood-lands are in full autumn foliage. Other mushrooms, such as the morels, spring up from rich soil in spring when the lilacs burst into bloom and apple trees are full of white blossoms. Still other mushrooms need the heat of summer and much rain before they will "mushroom." The most important factor affecting the fruit-ing of mushrooms is moisture. If there has been no rain in a region for a long time, few if any mushrooms will be found. However, if a soaking rain or a series of gentle rains occurs, the woodlands and fields may explode with fungi. Because mush-rooms sometimes seem to spring up overnight, the early Greeks thought that lightning bolts striking the ground during a rain-storm created the mushrooms.

The growth of a mushroom into maturity occurs when the existing cells in a knob or button on a mycelium suddenly fill with water and other material that have been absorbed from the soil. The cells stretch, and the mushroom "balloon" expands rapidly. In an amanita (Figure 1) this rapid elongation causes the cap to break through the outer covering of the button known as the universal veil. The veil breaks into pieces which may cling to the top of the cap. The rest of the veil remains at the bottom and forms a cup or *volva*. As the cap expands, the tissue that covers the area on which the gills are developing breaks apart and hangs on the stem as a *ring* or *annulus*. In the end, a mature fruiting body complete with *cap*, *gills*, and *stem* (*stipe*) forms.

The enormous strength of these expanding mushrooms is sur-prising. When the cells stretch, they act like tiny hydraulic rams that create a slow but steady pressure against any object above the growing mushroom. This steady pressure over a period of time is enough to weaken asphalt and to split concrete. Fruiting mush-rooms have been known to push their way up through a 3-inch-thick layer of asphalt, to lift wine casks in a winery high off a cellar floor, and to break through concrete floors in factories. In England, an 83-pound stone slab 2 feet in diameter was freed of its cement shackles and lifted 2 inches off the ground. When

British residents looked underneath the stone, they found what were probably two small meadow mushrooms balancing the stone in the center.

One of the most dramatic examples of mushroom power was described by Italian mycologists Augusto Rinaldi and Vassili Tyndalo in *The Complete Book of Mushrooms*. Some people in a courtyard heard a loud noise like an exploding firecracker coming from a portico that faced the courtyard. The concrete floor of the portico then split and rose into the air, revealing several compact agaric mushrooms in the floor opening.

Groups of Mushrooms

To propagate mushroom offspring, an interesting variety of methods for dispersing spores has evolved in the fruiting bodies. (Figure 2). In fact, mycologists use these methods of spore dispersal to divide fungi into major groups. The larger fungi form two major groups, the *Basidiomycetes* and the *Ascomycetes*. In the Basidiomycetes, the spores form on club-shaped cells called *basidia* (the Latin word for "clubs"). There are usually four spores to a basidium. In the Ascomycetes, the spores are normally found inside small cells or sacs, called *asci*. Four or eight spores are usually found in each ascus. Most of the larger fleshy fungi including the edible mushrooms are Basidiomycetes.

The agarics, or gilled fungi, are a common group of Basidiomycetes. The spores, as mentioned earlier, form on the gills of these mushrooms. In the boletes, instead of gills on the underside of the cap, a sponglelike layer of thin, vertical tubes is present. The spores form inside these tubes and exit through openings in the tube layer known as pores. With the exception of the tube layer, a bolete looks like a gilled mushroom that has a cap and stem.

In a third group of mushrooms (teeth fungi), teeth replace the gills or pore tubes underneath the cap, while in a fourth type of mushrooms (chanterelles), wrinkled veins are the spore-produc-

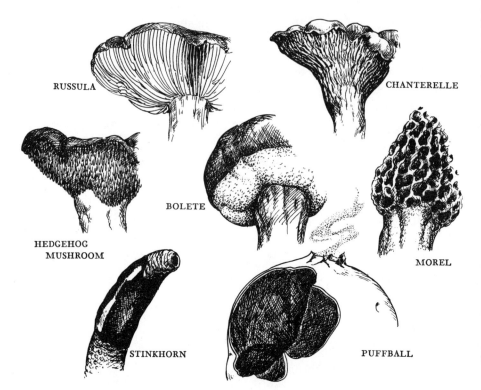

FIGURE 2. *Spores may be produced (beginning clockwise, top left) on gills, wrinkled surfaces, in pits, inside fungi, on an odor-bearing surface, on teeth, and (center) in pore tubes.*

ing surfaces. An example of the Ascomyetes is the delicious morel. Here the cap has a pitted, spongelike surface, and in the pits the surface is lined with spore-producing asci.

In all the mushrooms just mentioned, the spore-producing surface is on the outside of the fruiting body. In a group of mushrooms known as the *Gasteromycetes*, the spores are produced inside the fungus. The term *Gasteromycetes*, which includes the puffballs and their relatives, means "stomach fungi," a reference to the fact that the spores are produced within these fungi. The spores are released when the skin of the fungus breaks or splits open. A breath of wind or even a raindrop striking the puffball is enough to trigger the release of the mature spores.

A mushroom with a cap and stem is a simple device for releasing a large number of spores. The stem elevates the spore-producing surface above the material on which the mushroom is growing. And the underside of the cap provides a large surface area for the spores to be launched. A gilled mushroom is more efficient than the wrinkled surface of a chanterelle, because there is more spore-bearing surface on gills than on the more primitive wrinkles of a chanterelle.

Among other mushrooms, even more intriguing methods of spore dispersal can be found. In the aptly named stinkhorns, for example, spores are transplanted to new localities by insects that are attracted by the odor of the mushroom. The spores are located on a cap perched on a long stipe. When the insects crawl over the cap, they become covered with spores. The spores are carried to a new area when the insects fly away.

The Role of Fungi

Fungi play three basic roles in nature: they decompose various kinds of organic matter (*saprophytes*), attack living organisms (*parasites*), and co-exist in a mutually beneficial way with trees and other large plants by linking up with the roots of these plants (*mycorrhizae*). While green plants build up organic material, fungi break down or decompose what the plants have built up. If for some inexplicable reason all the fungi (and the closely related bacteria) in the world were to cease functioning, much of the land surface would soon be buried in plant and animal remains.

SAPROPHYTES Mushrooms that live on dead or decaying plant material are known as *saprophytes*. Saprophytic mushrooms can live on plant material as diverse as pine needles, broad leaves, dead limbs, and logs. Many of these mushrooms are so specialized that they will live only on certain types of material. This characteristic is an important clue when looking for edible mushrooms. For example, the aptly named meadow mushroom (*Agaricus campestris*), a close relative of the cultivated mushroom, lives only in meadows, fields, and on lawns; it feeds on nutrients provided by decaying grasses, manure (or lawn fertilizer), and other material. Because of its specialized needs, the meadow mushroom is never found growing in woodlands.

PARASITES   Parasitic fungi attack living plants. Some parasitic mushrooms are very destructive to forest trees. They may rot a tree's interior and cause millions of dollars worth of damage to commercial timber each year. The honey mushroom (*Armillariella mellea*), a popular edible fungus, attacks and kills the roots of oaks and other trees. Lines of this mushroom can sometimes be seen paralleling the roots of a tree. Clusters may also be seen smothering the base of a tree or its trunk. The tenacity of these parasitic fungi is impressive. I once saw a honey mushroom perform a delicate balancing act on a root projecting from a roadside cut across the street from my house. The root, exposed by erosion, was about a half inch in diameter. It was so close to the road that passing traffic caused the small root to bob up and down. Yet, despite its precarious position, the parasitic fungus clung, draining the tree to which the root belonged of its life processes.

Several fungi may be considered weak parasites because they only attack trees previously weakened by other factors such as disease or storm damage. In rare cases, one fungus will attack and parasitize another fungus. One species of boletes, for example, can be found only on the hard earthballs known as *Sclerodermas*.

MYCORRHIZAE   Not all mushrooms, of course, are harmful to living plants. In fact, scientists have discovered that a large group of mushrooms are actually beneficial to living trees. These fungi obtain food from the tree, while the tree, in turn, gets food with the help of the fungi. The first clue to this unusual relationship was uncovered in the late 1880s by the German scientist A. B. Frank. When Dr. Frank dug up trees, he found a sheath of fine hairs or threads surrounding the tiny roots of the trees. On some trees, the sheath of fungus threads completely surrounded the entire rootlet. In other cases, they penetrated the rootlets, yet did not seem to harm the tree. These fine threads, it eventually turned out, were linked to mushrooms on the surface.

Dr. Frank called the interrelationship between the mushroom threads and tree roots *mycorrhiza*, "fungus root." He correctly concluded that the mycorrhizal relationship is beneficial to both mushroom and the host tree. When mycorrhizae are present, trees seem to grow much faster and are healthier. The mushrooms, in turn, thrive on the food obtained from the trees. Remove the trees and you remove the mushroom's food supply.

More recently, researchers have obtained a clearer picture of just how beneficial this mycorrhizal relationship is to the participants. It has been found that a huge network of mycorrhizae surrounding a tree's root system acts much like the large net of a fisherman. Just as a larger net enables a fisherman to increase his catch, so does a large mycorrhizal network enable a tree to draw much larger amounts of phosphorus, water, and other material needed for growth into the root system. Much of this material would be lost if it weren't for the mycorrhizae. Thus mycorrhizae help a tree to grow even in very poor soil.

What does a fungus receive in return? A mushroom obtains carbon compounds, vitamins, and other food from root tissue. Some mushrooms have become so dependent on tree roots for food that they cannot survive by themselves. Many mushrooms will form mycorrhizae only with certain trees, another important identification clue for the mushroom gatherer. Certain edible boletes, for example, will grow only under pine trees; other boletes prefer birch trees. Some mycorrhizal fungi are less restrictive. The delicious yellow chanterelles may link up with the rootlets of many kinds of trees.

The list of mushrooms that form mycorrhizae with trees continues to increase. They include the boletes, the poisonous amanitas, the colorful russulas, and the milky lactarius mushrooms. Until recently, the saprophytic fungi seemed to be the most common mushrooms. However, as more mycorrhizal mushrooms are discovered, this group now seems to be almost as popular as the saprophytes.

Is It Edible or

Poisonous?

There are more than 5,000 fleshy kinds of mushrooms in the United States. Not only do they come in all shapes and sizes and grow in various habitats, but they also exhibit a remarkable range in edibility. Some, like the morel, are delicious; others are more bland tasting. There is also a large group of mushrooms that are considered inedible. Inedible does not necessarily mean poisonous. It may be that the mushroom is bitter or tasteless, or the fungus may be so small or so tough that it is not worth collecting. At the other end of the spectrum are the mushrooms that cause adverse, or poisonous, reactions in humans. Poisonous mushrooms vary considerably in their effects. In some cases, a mushroom may cause a brief stomach upset; a short time later, the afflicted person completely recovers. In other cases, a mushroom may be so toxic that eating one cap of the mushroom can cause death.

According to Gary Lincoff and D. H. Mitchel, authors of *Toxic and Hallucinogenic Mushroom Poisoning*, a handbook for physicians and mushroom hunters, "most mushroom poisonings occur from a limited number of kinds, perhaps a hundred species, of which fewer than a dozen are considered deadly." Most mushroom deaths in the United States are caused by eating the deadly false morels (*Gyromitra*), including a species that is widely collected and eaten in Europe and in the western part of the United States. This toxin, called *monomethylhydrazine* or MMH, is identical to a fuel propellent used in the U.S. space program. MMH, which is formed from another toxin in false morels, called *gyromitrin*, has caused some deaths. A third category includes the toxin *coprine*, a substance found in inky cap mushrooms—fungi that become inky when mature. Coprine has the unusual characteristic of being toxic only when mushrooms containing this toxin are consumed with alcoholic drinks. Though the symptoms of coprine poisoning—rapid pulse, flushed face, tingling of the arms and legs—may seem frightening to the uninitiated, the best antidote to this form of mushroom poisoning is simply "reassurance."

The fourth group contains toxins found in hallucinogenic mushrooms. Persons who ingest the hallucinogenic or "magic" mushrooms may question the placement of these mushrooms in the toxic category. However, Dr. Donald Simons, a mushroom toxicologist, considers "a toxin as anything that disrupts physiological processes in humans . . . whether or not a person eats a mushroom to achieve a desirable effect is irrelevant." In addition to the substances that cause hallucinogenic effects, toxic compounds have been found in certain hallucinogenic mushrooms that produce reactions that even magic-mushroom devotees would not consider desirable.

The final category of mushroom toxins is a broad grouping where toxins that primarily cause gastrointestinal upsets are lumped together. The symptoms generally do not last long, but can be disturbing. Recovery is typically rapid.

The Deadliest Mushrooms

Amanitas probably cause about 90 percent of all mushroom deaths in the United States and Europe. The mushroom most often blamed for the European deaths is the death cup (*Amanita phalloides*). The mushroom with the olive-green cap has the typical

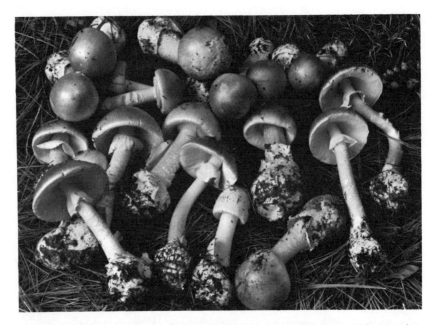

FIGURE 3. *There is probably enough poison in this group of amanitas* (Amanita phalloides) *to kill more than a dozen persons. The chief characteristics of deadly amanitas are very evident at various stages of growth.*

characteristics of an amanita (Figure 3): white gills, a skirtlike ring on the stipe, and a volva. Although the reported cases of deaths from amanitas usually involve individuals or family members who have mistakenly collected this mushroom, large groups may also be involved. The most tragic single incident of *Amanita phalloides* poisoning occurred near Poznań, Poland, in 1918, when thirty-one school children died after eating a dish of these mushrooms at school.

Although *Amanita phalloides* is predominantly a European mushroom, it has been recorded with increasing frequency in the United States. The mushroom is believed to have made the transatlantic jump some years ago, either by spores carried by air currents, or by spores or mycelia that were in the soil of plants imported into this country. This species has since gained a mycelial hold in the United States, being now found in the Northeast, in the Mid-Atlantic states, as far south as Virginia, and in the western part of the United States. In 1979, it was reported in Ohio for the first time. Already several deaths have been attributed to this mushroom in this country.

More commonly found in the United States are the related but equally deadly amanitas known as the destroying angels. The major difference between the destroying angels and the *Amanita phalloides* is the color of the cap. The destroying angels are entirely white, including the cap, while the *Amanita phalloides* is white except for its olive-green cap. There are six species of white amanitas known as the destroying angels. They are the *Amanitas verna, virosa, bisporigera, tenuifolia, suballiacea,* and *ocreata.* With the exception of *Amanita tenuifolia* and *Amanita suballiacea,* all of these destroying angels have been known to cause deaths in the United States.

Amanitas responsible for poisonings are often mistaken for other types of mushrooms. For example, in California, which has more serious or fatal cases of mushroom poisonings than any other state in western North America, the white *Amanita ocreata* or the green-capped *Amanita phalloides* has been mistaken for another amanita that is edible and commonly collected in California. This edible species, *Amanita calyptroderma,* is a large mushroom with an orange to orange-brown cap that is partially covered with a patch on top. In the past, most of the serious or fatal poisonings in California have been attributed to *Amanita phalloides,* a common species in that state. Now, however, a research team of Drs. Joseph F. Ammirati and Paul A. Horgen, both of the University of Toronto, and Harry D. Thiers of San Francisco State University have found that the white *Amanita ocreata* should also be held responsible. In a 1977 issue of *Mycologia,* the scientific journal of the Mycological Society of America, the scientists noted that over the years fatal cases of mushroom poisoning have been reported in California during the late winter and spring months, often after *Amanita phalloides* finished fruiting for the season. A study of the California amanitas revealed that both *Amanita calyptroderma* and *Amanita ocreata* commonly appeared in the spring. When the latter species was analyzed, toxins as deadly as those in *Amanita phalloides* were found. The scientists concluded that *Amanita ocreata* was, in fact, a deadly poisonous species and "probably caused some of the fatal cases of mushroom poisoning in California, especially those that occurred in the spring."

When a deadly amanita is eaten, the symptoms do not appear immediately. In fact, if a person quickly develops symptoms such as a stomach upset, it's most likely that the mushroom is not deadly. In amanita poisonings, the symptoms usually begin ten hours after the mushroom has been eaten, although they may occur as early as six hours or as late as twenty-four hours. The symptoms include severe abdominal pain, diarrhea, and vomiting. The symptoms usually last a day. Then, the person passes through a stage in which he seems to be improving. The victim, if in a hospital, may even be released from the hospital. However, the next stage is the critical stage. since the toxins have been steadily attacking the cells of the liver and kidneys. Even during the six to twenty-four hours before the initial symptoms were felt, the toxins were starting to destroy the liver and kidney cells. By the final stage, about the fourth day after the amanitas have been eaten, the liver and kidneys may fail and death will occur.

The fatal toxins in amanita poisonings are the *amatoxins*. These toxins are ten times deadlier than cyanide. Amatoxins, which include potent chemicals called amanitins, attack the nucleus of the liver cell and prevent the synthesis of protein, thereby destroying the cell. The toxins are also filtered out of the blood by the kidneys, and the cells in these organs are also attacked. Instead of passing out of the body through the kidneys, the amanitins may then be reabsorbed into the bloodstream and recirculated back to the liver, causing further damage. Another group of toxins called phallotoxins have also been found in amanitas. Although once considered extremely destructive, the phallotoxins are actually much less toxic than the amanitins and scientists now believe that these poisons play a small role, if any, in human amanita poisonings.

Recently, amanitins have been discovered in mushrooms other than amanitas. *Galerinas*—small, dingy brown mushrooms with long, thin, brittle stems that grow mostly in deep moss and on wood—may also contain toxic levels of amanitins. These small mushrooms are so unimpressive, you would think no one would be interested in gathering them. But severe poisoning, including at least one death, have been attributed to three species of *Galerina* in the United States. A fourth species, found in Japan, has caused several deaths. The three U.S. species include *Galerina autumnalis*, a mushroom that grows on logs in late fall, *Galerina venenata*, a rare mushroom found in grass in the Pacific Northwest, and *Galerina marginata*, which grows in dense clusters on rotten wood. About twenty of these small mushrooms are needed to produce a fatal reaction.

Amanitins are still being discovered in more mushrooms. The toxic levels range from large amounts found in another little brown mushroom (*Conocybe filaris*) to amounts so small that the amanitins do not produce any physiologic effect in humans. These more recent discoveries seem to suggest that the presence of amanitins may be normal in the development of a mushroom. However, for some reason, very large amounts of amanitins were produced in amanitas and *Galerinas* (or *Conocybe*) at some stage in their evolutionary development.

To the unknowing, the consumption of a deadly amanita can seem like an automatic death warrant. Yet people do survive after eating supposedly deadly amounts of amanitas. In fact, recent studies using new techniques of treating amanitin poisoning have been so successful that the survival rate in the many cases of at least one of these studies reached 100 percent!

One promising drug for treating amanita poisoning is thioctic acid. Thioctic acid occurs in many plants and animals, including humans. In the late 1950s, scientists reported that thioctic acid seemed to be effective in treating liver disease in animals. In 1964, Czech scientist Jiří Kubicka tried the substance on persons who had been poisoned by *Amanita phalloides*. When large doses were administered, the survival rate of these victims dramatically improved. In one set of experiments, thirty-nine out of forty patients survived after being treated with thioctic acid.

In the United States, nearly equal success was reported by Frederick C. Bartter of the National Heart and Lung Institute at the National Institutes of Health (NIH) in Bethesda, Maryland.

In twelve cases of persons suffering from amanitin poisoning who were treated between 1970 and 1975, eleven lived. In some cases, scar tissue, evidence of healing, was observed in the liver and kidneys. In treating amanitin poisoning, thioctic acid is used in conjunction with glucose (sugar). Patients are fed the glucose intravenously to counteract the effects of low blood sugar (hypoglycemia) produced by amanitin poisoning.

Thioctic acid has not yet been approved for general use in the United States. It is still considered an "investigative new drug" and is only available on special request from Dr. Bartter. However, any doctor with a patient who may have been poisoned by amanitins may call NIH at any hour of the day or night to request the drug (days: 301 496–6268; nights: 301 656–4000). It will then be dispatched by plane, state trooper, or even a helicopter, depending on which method is best in a given area. In the western part of the United States, thioctic acid can be obtained from Dr. Charles E. Becker, at Laguna Honda Hospital in San Francisco, California (phone number: 415 565–8324).

In England, British doctors have another method of treating *Amanita phalloides* poisoning. They remove the toxins by passing the blood through a device containing charcoal. When seven persons who had eaten lethal doses of amanitins were treated by this method, the vomiting and diarrhea rapidly subsided in all cases, and no signs of liver failure were observed. After only three days, four of the patients were well enough to leave the hospital. According to a recent report in *Lancet,* a British medical journal, the British doctors state that "our cases provide strong circumstantial evidence that charcoal can effectively remove toxins from the blood, even 24 hours after eating *Amanita phalloides.*"

And, finally, in another series of tests conducted in Europe, a 100-percent survival rate was achieved in thirty-three patients suffering from amanitin poisoning when large doses of penicillin were added to the doctor's repertoire for treating amanitin poisoning (glucose, thioctic acid, and other support measures). The penicillin was administered continuously each day within a day or two after *Amanita phalloides* was eaten. The penicillin seems to prevent amanitins from hitching a ride onto other substances that are recycled through the bloodstreams after passing through the kidneys. The amanitins pass out of the body from the kidneys without causing damage. Despite the high dosage of penicillin, no side effects have been noticed. And the treatment was extremely successful.

More studies will be needed before any of these antidotes can definitely be called a complete cure in treating amanitin poisoning; however, the preliminary results are encouraging.

Mushrooms with the Rocket-Fuel Poison

While conducting research in mushroom toxicology, scientists sometimes come upon cases that seem to defy explanation. No common mycelial thread seems to tie the cases together even though the same mushroom is implicated in the poisoning. Such is the case with the false morel, *Gyromitra esculenta*, also known as the brain mushroom or lorchel. This mushroom (see Color Plate 4) looks somewhat like a real morel except that the cap has brainlike folds, whereas the morels have a pitted or spongelike cap. Each spring, *Gyromitra esculenta* is widely sought as an edible in Europe as well as in some parts of the United States, especially in western North America. An estimated 1 million persons throughout the world eat this false morel each year, and gourmet shops often stack cans of *Gyromitra esculenta* on the shelves alongside cans of the famous and delicious real morel (*Morchella esculenta*). As an apparent vindication of the edibility of the false mushroom, even the Latin name of this species, *esculenta,* means "edible."

Yet for some reasons, persons have become ill or even died from eating the false morel. There are cases where one person became ill while eating *Gyromitra esculenta* even though several others at the same table were not affected. Or a person would feel fine one day; yet, if another batch of false morels were eaten the next day, serious illness or even death would result. There are even cases where a person became ill from inhaling the fumes from false morels that were cooking.

Why does this mushroom have such a varying effect? The answer was discovered quite by accident. In 1970, Donald Simons, a du Pont chemist in Wilmington, Delaware, was doing research for an article on mushroom toxins for the *Delaware Medical Journal*. In his research, Dr. Simons learned that two German scientists, P. H. List and P. Luft, had isolated a toxic chemical in the false morel that they called *gyromitrin*. This toxin, they found, breaks down into another deadly toxin called *monomethyl- hydrazine*, or MMH. This chemical is the same MMH that was used as rocket fuel to help send Apollo astronauts to the moon. "By a stroke of luck," recalled Dr. Simons, "while doing research in a library, I bumped into a physician at du Pont who had worked with MMH and who knew about some research being done on the substance at Wright-Patterson Air Force Base in Dayton, Ohio." The research, though it was not the intent of the Air Force scien- tists, yielded the long-sought answer to the mystery of why some mushroomers became ill or died from eating false morels while many, many more were not affected.

The original purpose of the Air Force experiments was to de- termine exactly how leaking rocket fuel affected the performance of technicians who were adding MMH propellent to the fuel chamber of rocket thrusters in the Apollo space capsule. MMH attacks the nervous system. It had already caused illness among the fuel handlers. Working with monkeys in the lab, Kenneth C. Back and Mildred K. Pinkerton found that at certain low levels monomethylhydrazine did not affect the animals. But if the ani- mals received higher doses on successive days, they became ill and eventually died. A very narrow limit was found in which MMH either produced no effect or caused sickness and death.

The research helped explain why one person became ill while eating the mushroom while others did not. The person who be- came ill ingested a higher level of MMH than the others. A person who became ill and died after eating mushrooms two days in a row went beyond the threshhold between the nontoxic level and a harmful or lethal level. "Perhaps many a gyromitra eater has run closer to the ragged edge than he realized," Dr. Simons noted in the *Delaware Medical Journal* article that he eventually wrote.

The typical symptoms of gyromitrin or MMH poisoning are similar to those of amanita toxins, but are experienced sooner. About six to eight hours after eating the mushrooms, there is a feeling of fullness in the stomach; vomiting, diarrhea, headaches, cramps, and abdominal pain follow. Liver damage and jaundice may also occur. In severe cases, convulsions, coma, and death result. In milder cases, the person recovers in one to three days. If so many people eat false morels, why is it that so few people become ill or die? The low death (or poisoning) rate is undoubtedly due to the widespread practice of boiling the mushroom for a long time in water and then throwing away the cooking liquid. It turns out that the toxin is soluble in water and will readily evaporate. Claims that a cook became ill while preparing the gyromitras while the diners experienced no effect is possible because the cook inhaled vapors containing volatile MMH. In some cases, however, even parboiling the mushrooms and discarding the water has failed to eliminate all of the toxins, and illness has resulted.

Gyromitrin may possibly be present in other *Gyromitra* or false morels; in some species, no toxin has been found. Recently it has been shown that MMH causes cancer in animals. In experiments at the Eppley Institute for Research in Cancer in Omaha, Nebraska, MMH and other chemical compounds derived from it (some of which occur in the false morel) cause liver and intestinal tumors in animals. However, no proof exists that eating the mushroom can cause cancer in humans. Yet to be perfectly safe from gyromitrin, MMH, or any possible carcinogen, no gyromitra species should be eaten.

Mixing Mushrooms with Alcohol

The phrase "If you drive, don't drink" crops up frequently to dissuade revelers from having accidents while driving home after a celebration. For some people who eat certain wild mushrooms, this phrase has to be modified to "If you eat inky caps and some other mushrooms, don't drink." The particular inky cap in question is *Coprinus atramentarius*, a gray mushroom (Figure 33) that grows in clumps in grass, around decaying trees, and almost anywhere on organic debris. It fruits most frequently in spring and fall during cool, wet weather. Some people have found, to their dismay, that when they imbibe alcohol a few hours after eating this mushroom, some surprising symptoms occur. Within ten to thirty minutes, the face and neck may flush, the heart begins to beat rapidly, a metallic taste is detected, the hands feel as if they are swelling, the arms and legs tingle, and the head feels light. Usually nausea and vomiting follow. With this brace of symptoms, no wonder the victims become alarmed. Yet, in most cases no treatment other than reassurance is required. The symptoms usually fade in a half hour to two hours.

The above symptoms are similar to those produced by disulfiram or Antabuse, a drug given to alcoholics to cure them of their desire to drink. After experiencing these reactions a few times, the alcoholic is likely to curb the temptation to drink. In 1975, a compound that causes the Antabuselike symptoms was isolated from *Coprinus atramentarius*. The compound, called *coprine*, was discovered almost simultaneously by researchers in Sweden and in the United States.

Coprine interrupts the process in which the liver breaks down or metabolizes the alcohol from an alcoholic drink. Normally, alcohol is changed in the liver into a chemical called acetaldehyde. This chemical is then converted into acetic acid, which in turn breaks down into carbon dioxide and water. However, coprine slows down the ability of the liver to convert the acetaldehyde to acetic acid. When acetaldehyde accumulates in the body in large enough amounts, it then stimulates the nervous system and produces the symptoms associated with inky cap poisoning.

Surprisingly, many people who consume alcohol along with the inky cap *Coprinus atramentarius* are not affected. I attended a meeting on mushroom toxicology at the Boston Mycological Club (BMC), where the various participants vigorously debated the effect of the mushroom-alcohol combination. Some people claimed that they had consumed alcohol with the mushroom for years and had never been affected. Others, however, described the frightening temporary effects of a bout with *Coprinus atramentarius* and alcohol.

For those who are sensitive, the time interval and the order of drinking and eating seem nearly as important, or even more important, than the amount of alcohol and mushrooms consumed. If a person has eaten the mushrooms before drinking alcohol, the symptoms can be as rapid as when an alcoholic takes an Antabuse pill. How long the reaction lasts depends on the level of alcohol in the blood. Some reports indicate that reactions may occur four or five days later whenever alcohol is drunk. Generally, no reactions will occur if only one drink is taken one or two hours before the mushrooms are eaten. However, three or four drinks within an hour of the mushroom feast may cause a reaction. Why some people are affected by eating this mushroom while others are not is still unknown.

In addition to *Coprinus atramentarius*, coprine has been found in three other species of inky caps in North America by George M. Hatfield of the University of Michigan. However, these species are not very common in the United States. The most common inky caps are *Coprinus atramentarius*, the glistening inky cap (*Coprinus micaceus*), and the shaggy-mane mushroom (*Coprinus comatus*). Although all three are collected for the table, the shaggy-mane is considered the choicest find and is extremely delicious. Fortunately, neither the shaggy-mane nor the glistening inky cap contain coprine, says Dr. Hatfield after an extensive analysis of North American inky caps for coprine. Some European books, however, claim that the glistening inky cap and the shaggy-mane have caused Antabuselike reactions in Europe. Is it possible that coprine is found only in the European species? Whatever the conclusion, beginners in the United States should limit themselves when eating inky caps to the shaggy-mane mushroom because it is so easily recognized and is one of the finest tasting mushrooms.

A similar reaction with alcohol has also been reported in persons who have eaten the club-footed clitocybe (*Clitocybe clavipes*). Cases of Antabuselike reaction have been reported in Michigan, Massachusetts, and New Jersey as well as in Japan when this mushroom was consumed with alcohol.

Other mushrooms can cause an upset when eaten before or after drinking alcohol. The symptoms in these cases differ from the typical inky cap reaction; essentially nausea and vomiting are the main symptoms. What causes these upsets is not known. One of the offenders has been the highly prized black morel (*Morchella angusticeps*). When eating this morel, it is best to avoid alcohol. Some people would even broaden this alcoholic ban to include other morels.

The Hallucinogenic Mushrooms

In the 1950s, when many young people were experimenting with LSD and other drugs, articles about hallucinogenic mushrooms began appearing in various publications. One of the most popular articles appeared in *Life* magazine in 1957 and was written by R. G. Wasson, a retired banker who has been fascinated for many years with the history of mushroom usage in various cultures, and who has helped pioneer a new interest in the area of ethnomycology. Wasson wrote about his experiences in Mexico, where he observed various "magic" mushrooms used by Indians in sacred ceremonies to obtain visions. He even tried some of the mushrooms to confirm the hallucinogenic experiences described by the Indians. When it was learned that some of these same mushrooms grew in fields in the United States, especially along the Gulf Coast, these open areas in the coastal states began filling up with youth who although they did not know a morel from a cultivated mushroom, did want to find some magic mushrooms.

In the 1970s, the search for these mushrooms increased when a wide variety of books and articles on hallucinogenic mushrooms appeared. Written mostly by amateurs, and often inaccurately, these publications extolled the merits of hallucinogenic mushrooms, pointing out how to identify and even cultivate these fungi. Some entrepeneurs, capitalizing on the interest in these mushrooms, have even offered to send spores of hallucinogenic mushrooms by mail.

The hallucinogenic mushrooms are small and inconspicuous and belong to the genera *Psilocybe, Panaeolus,* and *Conocybe.* To find *Psilocybe* mushrooms, searchers rely on only two key field characteristics: they grow on or near dung in pastures and have stems that turn blue when handled. This color change has resulted in the popular name "blue legs" for at least one species. Because even scientists have difficulty identifying these little brown mushrooms, amateurs may mistakenly choose another mushroom and become severely poisoned.

In 1958, at the Sandoz Pharmaceutical Laboratories in Switzerland, a research team lead by Dr. Albert Hofmann, the same scientist who synthesized LSD, identified the two chemicals that cause the hallucinogenic effects. The chemicals, called *psilocybin* and *psilocin,* were obtained from mushrooms grown in the laboratory from material that had been collected in Mexico. Psilocybin changes chemically into psilocin, which, in turn, oxidizes into a blue substance. The bluing is the same bluing seen in the stems of psilocybe mushrooms.

The effects of eating hallucinogenic mushrooms can be quite spectacular, judging by the descriptions given by such disparate individuals as Mexican Indians, R. G. Wasson, college students, members of the street scene, and even Carlos Castaneda, the author of best-selling books about the teachings of an Indian sorcerer whom he calls Don Juan. Most experiences seem pleasant, although some can be bad.

Within thirty to sixty minutes after hallucinogenic mushrooms are eaten, a person may feel pleasant or apprehensive (a "good" or a "bad" trip). Sharp outlines of objects, brilliant colors, and a variety of scenes are visualized when the eyes are closed. During the second hour, colors become more intense and brilliant, often forming various patterns, such as a burst of fireworks. These patterns are sometimes superimposed on dreamlike shapes that rapidly appear and disappear. These visions continue for another hour, and then gradually disappear. Unlike the drug alcohol, no hangover symptoms occur after the experience.

Not all experiences are necessarily pleasurable. Nausea and vomiting may occur, even temporary paralysis. On a bad trip, persons have panicked and experienced fears of death or insanity. They found it difficult to distinguish the real world from fantasy. These mushrooms can lead to convulsions and death in young children.

Gastrointestinal Irritants

The list of mushrooms that cause gastrointestinal upsets (vomiting or diarrhea or both) is large. They include representatives from many groups such as the milky caps (*Lactarius*), russulas, coral mushrooms, and the boletes. The toxins are often difficult to identify, and the symptoms, which may appear rapidly (within fifteen minutes to four hours), usually do not last long. The second word in the name of this category, "irritant," aptly describes the situation of a person who eats a mushroom containing a toxin that causes these primarily irritating symptoms.

Like the inky cap, many mushrooms in this group seem to affect only certain people. In fact, the percentage may sometimes be so small that the question arises: When is a case simply an idiosyncratic reaction of one individual, and when does it actually involve a toxin that would affect many people? Just as you will find someone, somewhere, who is very sensitive to strawberries, so too will there be some persons who are sensitive to certain mushrooms. Thousands of people may eat the cultivated mushroom each day without suffering any side effects, but one person who is sensitive to this edible fungus may have a strong reaction.

Among wild mushrooms, there are several species that are very selective in their effects. An example of a mushroom that causes gastrointestinal irritation only to certain persons is *Gomphus floccosus*. In older books on mushrooms, this shaggy, horn-shaped mushroom is sometimes listed as edible, and at other times as poisonous. The reason for this confusion is that many people eat this mushroom without experiencing any problem. Yet some others report digestive upsets. The principal toxin believed responsible, when these reactions do occur, has been segregated. It is *norcaperatic acid*, a substance that is structurally similar to citric acid, which is commonly found in oranges, grapefruits, and other citric fruits. The toxin also causes digestive upsets when two other species of *Gomphus* are eaten.

Recently, scientists have discovered that the edibility of a mushroom may also depend on the area where it is found. A mushroom may be widely collected and edible in most parts of the country, but in one region, it may cause a mild stomach upset. The very popular edible mushroom, the chicken mushroom or sulphur shelf, may be an example of this. This brightly colored fungus is considered one of the best edibles in North America and has been eaten with impunity for many years. Yet, in California, seven mild cases of mushroom poisoning were reported in which persons became nauseous and vomited after eating the mushroom either raw or cooked. The symptoms did not last long. Not all persons eating the mushrooms at these meals were affected, which could indicate differences in individual sensitivity. However, Thomas J. Duffy and Paul P. Vergeer in *California Toxic Fungi* believe that the results "suggest the occurrence of local mildly toxic forms." Dr. Donald Simons has another explanation for the problems produced by the sulphur shelf. He thinks some people's systems have trouble digesting chitin, a hard substance found in the cell walls of the *Polyporus sulphureus*. Because chitin swells in an alkaline environment such as in the intestines, gastrointestinal problems could result from eating a lot of sulphur shelf mushrooms rich in chitin. Thus the problem may be a matter of roughage, rather than that of being due to a toxin. Perhaps, this problem could be reduced in sensitive persons by limiting themselves to eating only the most tender parts of the sulphur shelf. In any case, it is always best the first time to sauté and sample only a small part of a mushroom before proceeding on to a larger repast.

While some mushrooms are delicious cooked, they may cause stomach upsets when eaten raw. In general, wild mushrooms should only be eaten cooked. (The few exceptions, such as the meadow mushroom, will be noted in Part II when the mushrooms are discussed in more detail.) There are enough ways of cooking mushrooms without needing to eat them raw.

Some cases of mushroom poisonings in which gastrointestinal symptoms are involved may be due to eating mushrooms that were too old and spoiled. Just as you wouldn't eat spoiled lettuce or overripe tomatoes, so too should very old mushrooms be avoided. In a two-year study of mushroom poisonings in Switzerland, researchers discovered that 20 percent of all reported poisonings resulted from eating spoiled "edible" mushrooms.

Other Toxins

Another group of toxins that scientists often categorize is the muscarine group. The toxin muscarine was the first mushroom poison to be identified. Originally extracted from *Amanita muscaria* or the fly agaric, the familiar reddish-capped mushroom illustrated in fairly tales, this toxin was once blamed for all mushroom poisonings. Some medical textbooks still perpetuate this error. Researchers have found that the fly agaric actually contains a miniscule amount of muscarine and that other toxins in that mushroom cause adverse reactions. Muscarine is actually found in larger quantities in small mushrooms that grow on lawns and paths (*Clitocybe dealbata*) and along shrub borders (*Inocybe* species). Muscarine stimulates the nervous system and causes various glands to work overtime. Tear ducts shed many tears, sweat glands produce much perspiration, and salivary glands salivate. Other signs and symptoms may include contraction of the pupils, a slowdown in the heartbeat, and a drop in blood pressure. The antidote that is effective against muscarine poisoning is atropine, a drug derived from the deadly nightshade (belladonna), a tall Eurasian plant with bell-shaped purple flowers.

Some cases of mushroom poisoning are not related to poisons produced by the mushrooms themselves. In 1975, a Massachusetts woman gathered edible mushrooms along a roadside and became poisoned after eating the mushrooms. The symptoms were those of lead poisoning. The toxins were discovered to have been deposited on the mushroom caps from exhaust fumes of passing cars burning leaded gasoline. A local neurologist warned against collecting mushrooms along busy thoroughfares as well as in areas that have been sprayed with pesticides or other toxic sprays. The warning continues to be applicable.

The Future of Mushroom Toxicology

Although mushroom toxicology is still considered a young science, much has been learned so that cases of mushroom poisoning can be accurately diagnosed (provided that the doctor has the necessary information). To achieve that goal, various mycological societies are working closely with local poison control centers or hospitals by supplying the names of mushroomers who can identify mushrooms suspected of poisoning or by publishing booklets that summarize the various categories of mushroom poisoning, including the mushroom characteristics, symptoms, and methods of treatment. A newly developed poison index is now also available for use in poison control centers in the United States. This index, which is stored on microfilm and updated every six months, includes information about the symptoms and treatment of mushroom poisoning as well as any other known poisoning. Another significant step in mushroom toxicology was achieved in 1977 when the book *Toxic and Hallucinogenic Mushroom Poisoning,* a handbook for physicians and mushroom hunters, was published. Written by Gary Lincoff, an amateur mycologist, and D. H. Mitchel, a physician, the book provides a comprehensive guide to the treatment of various types of mushroom poisoning. However, if you educate yourself and practice reasonable caution, you should never have to receive such treatment.

American Mushroom Gatherers: Past and Present

No scribe was present to record the event, but the first person to eat an edible wild mushroom in North America was undoubtedly an ancestor of today's American Indian. Many thousands of years ago Paleo-Indian women and their children may have been gathering edible wild plants, nuts, and berries while the men were hunting or fishing, when one of the women spotted a large clump of an interesting looking fungus. The mushrooms may have been a cluster of golden chanterelles or boletes beckoning from the dark recesses of a stand of evergreens. Or, perhaps, they were delectable morels. Whatever the species, the woman probably decided to add the fungi to the coffer of wild edibles collected that day for the evening meal.

Of course, the Paleo-Indian woman had no way of knowing whether or not the mushroom was edible. Such knowledge had to be obtained through the traditional method of trial and error. If a person did not get sick eating a particular wild food for the first time and the item tasted good, then it became part of the diet. All knowledge of the edibility of wild foods was probably garnered in this way. Once obtained, this information was passed on from generation to generation.

From this inauspicious beginning, a rich tradition of eating edible wild mushrooms sprang up in the Indian culture. Edible mushrooms became a staple food among such disparate Indian groups as the Plains Indians, the Indians of California, the Hopis and other tribes of the arid Southwest, and the woodland Indians of the East. The tradition became firmly established, and anthropologists who studied various Indian tribes in the late 1800s and early 1900s noted that wild mushrooms were still an important part of the Indian diet.

The descendants of the Iroquois Indians, a powerful league of tribes in the Northeast, told anthropologist A. C. Parker, himself an Indian, that the Iroquois ranked the pleasure of eating wild mushrooms as virtually equal to that of eating meat. The Iroquois favored several kinds of mushrooms, including the meadow mushrooms, puffballs, and morels. The meadow mushroom was favored by other tribes as well.

The elders of the Indian tribes also had many stories to tell about the ancient uses of the edible fungi. The Iroquois made soup from mushrooms. The mushrooms were peeled, cut into small pieces, and thrown into boiling water seasoned with salt and animal grease. Sometimes bits of meat were added to the soup.

Large quantities of mushrooms were dried by some Indian tribes to be used later for food. Matilda Cox Robinson, who accompanied her anthropologist husband during a stay among the Zuñi Indians of the Southwest in 1879, recounted how Indians gathered puffballs in great numbers. Although some of these puffballs were eaten immediately, many were dried for winter use. White settlers apparently took their cue from the Indians because they too ate puffballs when they went West. Puffballs were also an important part of the wild medicine cabinet of American Indians. Many tribes found that the spongy puffball acted as a dressing and effectively stopped the bleeding of cuts and deeper wounds. Puffball powder (actually the spores) was also sprinkled on wounds. The powder acted as a styptic, causing the blood vessels to contract.

The attitude that the North American Indian had toward mushrooms was most likely not shared by the white settlers who came over from Europe in the seventeenth century. Most of the early settlers in the American colonies came from Great Britain. Settling Virginia, Massachusetts, and other colonies, the Anglo-Saxons brought with them an attitude toward wild mushrooms— unbridled fear—that has largely persisted in the United States to this day. The British considered nearly all mushrooms poisonous, and derisively called them toadstools. This term arose from an old belief that toads were poisonous, and a typical cap of a mushroom seemed to be an ideal stool or resting place for the toads. The British fear of mushrooms was so intense that one irritated nineteenth-century British mycologist called the phobia a "national trait."

During the early hard times on the American continent, the colonists willingly allowed the Indians to teach them how to plant corn, stalk game, and eat certain wild greens. But the early settlers apparently drew the line when it came to eating wild mushrooms, and the fear seems to have persisted. A weathered gravestone at Trinity Episcopal Church in the Hudson River Valley town of Peekskill, New York, tells a grim story. The barely readable inscription recounts the death of William Gould, thirty-five, his wife Sarah, thirty-four, and their four-year-old son Charles. These "natives of the town of Noth. Wotton, England," according to the inscription, were "Poisoned by Eating Fungi (Toadstools)" The deaths occurred on October 2, 1838. This tombstone inscription is the oldest known *written* record of a death from mushroom poisoning in the United States.

The British mushroom phobia did not apply to all mushrooms. The British were especially fond of one type of mushroom, the cultivated white mushroom. This mushroom, which had been cultivated in England and France since the late 1600s, was also grown in colonial gardens, according to early records. Recipes for preparing the cultivated fungus appear in eighteenth-century cookbooks published in the United States. Thomas Jefferson recalled seeing the cultivated mushroom in the Washington, D.C., market when he was president. Jefferson, known for his lavish entertaining and appreciation of fine foods, used to arise early to visit the market and assist his servants in selecting the food for the day. He would keep a detailed record of the earliest and latest appearance of each vegetable in the Washington market. A chart published in Thomas Jefferson's *Garden Book*, a collection of his agricultural observations, showed that the earliest appearance of the white mushrooms over an eight-year period was August 11, the latest October 19.

The cultivated mushroom was grown from a starter material imported from England. The starter material, called *spawn* by professional mushroom growers, was actually mycelia of the cultivated mushroom that had permeated dried or flaky manure. When the spawn was added to beds in colonial gardens, white mushrooms appeared in summer and fall.

Early American settlers from countries other than Britain may not have shared the British caution toward wild mushrooms. One such ethnic group were the Germans. Most Germans settled in Pennsylvania; others went to New York and New Jersey. Germans were so numerous in Pennsylvania that Benjamin Franklin estimated, just before the American Revolution, that one-third of the Pennsylvania population came from Germany. Because some parts of Germany have a rich tradition of eating wild mushrooms, some of the German colonists probably gathered wild mushrooms.

Gradually, the taste for mushrooms spread. Orson K. Miller, Jr., author of the comprehensive mushroom identification book *Mushrooms of North America*, has evidence that early settlers in the mountains of Maryland and Virginia (many of Germanic descent) ate wild mushrooms. "I have talked to elderly people (in the mountains) who can remember a long history of spring gathering of morels in their families," recalls Dr. Miller. He thinks that the parents and grandparents of these people "would easily reach back to settlement times in the 1820–1850 period." Dr. Miller also suspects "that in almost every case, mushroom use was a combination of knowledge brought from Europe and augmented by knowledge gained from the North American Indians."

In the 1860s during the Civil War many southerners suddenly found themselves eating wild mushrooms in order to survive. The war had a devastating impact on the South. Most of the battles took place in that region, and the land bore the scars. Large areas were in ruin, thousands of farms were abandoned, many cities were bombarded or gutted by fire, and crops were destroyed. Food was scarce, and starvation threatened many sections. As the poet Sidney Lanier wrote the year the Civil War ended, "Pretty much the whole of life has been merely not dying."

To many southerners "merely not dying" meant living off the land. Wild foods, including mushrooms, were eaten. The Reverend M. A. Curtis, an eminent nineteenth-century botanist and collector of wild mushrooms, observed that many people in the southern states "found fungi of great importance to them" during the latter part of the Civil War. Curtis himself, a resident of Wilmington, North Carolina, eventually was forced to focus his energies on gathering "edible mushrooms from which I have gotten many a substantial and luxurious meal." After sharing his knowledge of mushrooms with other southerners, the botanist decided to write a book on identifying edible wild mushrooms. Unfortunately the book that he wrote, *Mycophagia Americana* ("Eating American Mushrooms"), was never published. During wartime, lamented Curtis, the cost of publishing such a book was too prohibitive. Years later, when the South recovered and food was once again plentiful, the habit of gathering wild mushrooms was probably largely abandoned.

In the latter half of the nineteenth century, a major event in the history of U.S. mycophagy occurred: the great migration of mushroom-loving immigrants to the United States from eastern and southern Europe. Starting as a trickle just after the Civil War and swelling to a flood in the last decade of the nineteenth century and the first two decades of the twentieth century, millions of persons poured into the United States from Italy, Poland, Russia, and Austria-Hungary. They crowded into Chicago, Detroit, Milwaukee, and other cities. They worked in the mines of Pennsylvania, and textile factories of New England, and on the farms of New Jersey. By 1921, when Congress passed a law restricting immigration from these countries, more than 11 million persons had entered the United States from Italy and from the Slavic countries.

One of the more interesting facets of the culture of these

peoples was their love of wild mushrooms and their custom of gathering them for the table. Back in the "old country," collecting and eating wild mushrooms was a time-honored, pleasant, and sometimes necessary tradition. Since childhood, the Poles, Russians, and Italians had been taught to distinguish between edible and poisonous mushrooms. They could distinguish the bolete from the morel, the chanterelle from the puffball, and the meadow mushrooms from the deadly amanita as easily as other people could distinguish a blueberry from a strawberry. The edible mushrooms were prepared in a multitude of ways for immediate use or pickled in barrels or dried on long strings over a stove for later use.

When these immigrants from eastern and southern Europe settled in the United States, they found to their delight that familiar species in the old country were also common here. The mushrooms were called by different names, but to the new Americans they were still *borowiki, maslaki,* or *porcini.*

Many of the edible mushrooms that the New Americans collected were known to all the eastern and southern European cultures; however, some species were more traditionally collected in one country or region than another. As a result, one could almost tell what country a person came from by the kind of mushrooms that were picked. A fellow mushroom gatherer, in the woods of Litchfield, Connecticut, once solemnly told me that in his area "The Russians pick the white mushrooms, the Poles the red mushrooms, and the Italians the brown mushrooms." Another example of this mycological dictum took place in the woods of my home town. During my father's many mushroom-gathering forays, he would often meet Jimmy, a small Italian American who lived in a nearby village. Jimmy would be searching for certain kinds of mushroom, my father for entirely different types. Whenever Jimmy saw what my father had in his brown bag, he would exclaim: "You eat those? You'd never catch me eating those things."

My father expressed equal horror at Jimmy's choices. The two men, with brown bag or basket in hand, would then continue on their separate ways. Two cultures, one Slavic the other Roman, had met in the woods of a new country and did not mingle. One day, my father invited Jimmy to the house to sample some of the mushrooms he had picked. After some hesitation, Jimmy agreed. When he ate the mushrooms, splendidly prepared by my mother, Jimmy's face creased with delight. He thought from then on that he would only pick the "Polish" mushrooms. I never did ask my father if he tried one of Jimmy's species.

The influence of the newest immigrants became discernible in the local markets of many towns and cities as wild mushrooms started appearing for sale. Meadow mushrooms, morels, and even puffballs vied for space with apples, carrots, turnips, and lettuce. This practice remains today in some cities where strings (or bags) of dried wild mushrooms gathered in Poland and other European countries can still be found in the stores of established ethnic neighborhoods. Imported canned wild mushrooms also appear in these stores as well as in specialty shops. In some states fresh wild mushrooms may still be seen for sale. In Boston, for example, the hen of the woods (*Polyporus frondosus*) may sometimes appear in a market in the Italian section, whereas in Michigan and in a few other states, fresh wild puffballs can still be found in farmers' markets. In the spring, in small country stores in the Midwest, freshly gathered morels are also sold.

At about the same time that large numbers of eastern and southern Europeans were arriving on the Atlantic side of the United States, much smaller groups of Japanese and Chinese were crossing the Pacific to settle in California and the Pacific Northwest. The Oriental immigrants also brought a rich tradition of enjoying mushrooms. Wild mushrooms have been important to Japanese and Chinese cuisine for countless generations. They are held in such high esteem that many species have also been cultivated.

Chinese immigrants relied primarily on dried and canned versions of their favorite mushrooms imported from the Orient. The Japanese newcomers on the other hand searched the woods for mushrooms similar to those found in Japan. In the early 1900s Japanese immigrants were frequently seen combing the pine and other evergreen woods in Washington and Oregon for the matsutake, or pine mushroom, a great delicacy in Japan. Although the true matsutake did not grow there, a close relative—a stocky, brownish-white mushroom with a pleasant, spicy odor—was discovered. The Japanese called this American mushroom the white matsutake. Scientists call it by the Latin name, *Armillaria ponderosa.*

The mushroom was very common in the Pacific Northwest. In the 1920s, C. H. Kaufman, a U.S. mycologist, observed that the mushroom was "common enough to be assiduously collected by the Japanese for commercial purposes." Today, second- and third-generation descendants of the original settlers still collect the mushroom and send white matsutakes to friends and relatives in California and in other areas where the mushroom does not grow.

Around the beginning of the twentieth century, interest in wild edible mushrooms began to spread to nonimmigrants as well. The Boston Mycological Club (BMC), the first amateur group of mushroom collectors in the Western Hemisphere, was formed in 1895. With the intent "to arouse a wider appreciation of the value of an abundant food which is, in America, comparatively neglected," the BMC conducted field trips and presented lectures on preparing and preserving mushrooms at the Massachusetts Horticultural Society's headquarters in Boston. The cooking demonstrations were quite impressive. Each affair included mushroom dishes ranging from soups and hors d'oeuvres to entrees and even desserts. A typical bill of fare presented by a Mrs. Annie Doughty in the late 1890s had eleven different mushroom dishes such as "purée aux oréades" (a mushroom soup of dried boletes and chanterelles), an entree of "fricasée aux cèpes" (boletes), and a dessert of "canapés à la Rothschild" (truffles and anchovies). The location of the Boston Mycological Club's headquarters, across the street from Music Hall where the world-famous Boston Symphony played, was a boon to many of its foreign-born musicians, who enjoyed eating wild mushrooms. These musicians would rush across the street before rehearsals with a batch of New World mushrooms they had collected for a quick identification and to enjoy delectable mushroom dishes.

The collecting of wild mushrooms during the early 1900s was not confined to immigrants or BMC members. In a 1914 issue of *Mycologia,* William Ford and Ernest Clark noted that "mushroom collecting has become something of a fad in many of our summer resorts . . . during September and October, the fields and pastures are pretty thoroughly searched for such species as the meadow mushroom, *Agaricus campestris*." They added that the mushroom hunters had learned to identify mushrooms with great accuracy.

Interest in wild mushrooms accelerated after World War II, when American servicemen returning from Europe discovered they had a more adventuresome palate than before the war. The recent interest in natural foods has also contributed to an increasing appreciation of wild mushrooms. As a result, more and more mushroom hunters are heading for nearby woodlands and fields to join descendants of settlers from Europe and Asian countries. Classes in mushroom identification at universities and colleges are overflowing and have long waiting lists. Mushroom clubs are springing up in different parts of the country. In Connecticut alone, three mushroom clubs now exist; a few years ago, none could be found. One club, the Puget Sound Mycological Society in the state of Washington, has more than 1,000 members.

On July 17, 1975, the status of mushrooms reached a "celestial zenith" that may never be surpassed, when American astronauts aboard the Apollo spececraft linked up with cosmonauts in the Soyuz vehicle, about 140 miles above the earth. During this historic alliance in space, U.S. astronauts Donald K. Slayton, Vance Brand, and Thomas Stafford shared with their Soviet counterparts an American lunch that included steak, grapefruit juice, strawberries, pears, apricots, and, you guessed it, mushroom soup. It is ironic that the Americans, and not the Russians, with their rich Slavic history of dining on mushrooms, offered mushroom soup. However, the U.S. astronauts were simply carrying on the tradition of some much earlier Americans, the American Indian.

In Pursuit of
Mushrooms

While twentieth-century technology has advanced many hobbies, sports, and other spare-time activities with such products as fiberglass fishing rods and powerful bird-watching scopes, equipment for the amateur mycologist has changed little over the years. Collecting mushrooms is still inexpensive and easy. A basket and a knife (and, of course, this guide) are all that most collectors of edible mushrooms will need. Two concessions that might be made to technology are a small magnifying lens for closeup views and the use of waxed paper to separate species.

BASKET.   On trips with mycological groups, I always see a wide variety of baskets. Some people prefer a small basket for ease of handling; others prefer a larger size, although there are people who note that "you usually don't find any mushrooms if you take a big basket." The basket I use is about 1 foot long, 10 inches wide, and 7 inches deep. Some people favor a basket with a lid to protect the mushrooms from rain and other material; but a lid can be awkward when you are handling mushrooms. In my youth, whenever I went mushroom collecting with my father, we always took a brown bag. We would fill the bag with boletes and bring them home for my mother to prepare a delicious meal. I have since graduated to a basket, because the different species can be kept separate more easily and the mushrooms are less apt to be squashed.

KNIFE.   A knife, preferably a hunting knife, is another important item. The knife enables you to remove mushrooms from wood easily, to dig out entire mushrooms, including the base, from the ground—to make sure you don't have an amanita—and to help you clean edible mushrooms on the spot. The knife can be kept in the basket or in a sheath on a belt.

WAX PAPER.   Wax paper is handy for separating different species of mushrooms. I carry a few large sheets of wax paper folded up in the basket as well as many wax sandwich bags. The smaller bags are good for storing a few mushrooms of a particular species. The larger collections can be placed between two sheets of wax paper; by twisting the ends of the sheets, you can store the mushrooms conveniently. Do not use plastic bags or plastic wrap. Mushrooms spoil rapidly inside plastic; the plastic enclosures are an ideal environment for bacteria.

You can place a slip of paper identifying the mushrooms in the wax bag containing the mushrooms or between wax sheets if you have a larger batch of mushrooms. Then, when you get home, you can study the mushrooms in a more leisurely way.

HAND LENS.   For closeup views of mushrooms, I carry a hand lens, a small magnifying glass that tucks into a small, hard, protective case when not in use. This tiny lens, about an inch long, magnifies mushroom features seven to ten times. The lens can be hung from your neck on a string or tied to the handle of your basket. Although nearly all of the identifying features of mushrooms in this book are easily seen with the naked eye, the hand lens is a definite aid in studying mushrooms close up and learning more about fungi. The lens may be purchased in hobby shops or from scientific supply houses such as Edmund Scientific Company Edscorp Building, Barrington, New Jersey 08007.

NOTEBOOK. I keep notes of my mushroom trips during the collecting season. Such data as what edible mushrooms were found, where, when, and the weather conditions are noted. After doing this for many years, I can look back in my little black book to find out when a certain mushroom usually first appears and what mushrooms I should expect to find during a particular month.

SPORE PRINTS. Obtaining a spore print is a valuable way of double-checking the identity of a species of mushroom. A spore print is not needed to identify such obvious species as morels or the sulphur shelf mushroom. But, for peace of mind, you may want to obtain a spore print of a meadow mushroom or an oyster mushroom. If so, insert 3 × 5 inch sheets of plain paper from a small pad inside a few of the wax paper bags before a collecting expedition. When you find a meadow mushroom for instance, you will note that the mushroom is white, stocky, has no cuplike base, has pink to brown gills, and grows in grass. But you may want to check that the spores are also brown. To make the spore print, simply cut the cap from the top of the stem. Insert the cap in a sandwich bag containing the sheet of paper, with the gill side down. Close the bag and place it in the basket face down. Meanwhile, collect several of the mushrooms that you have tentatively identified, and separate them from other species by storing them in wax paper bags. By the time you return from your foray, you should have a brown spore print on the paper in your sandwich bag that will definitely confirm your find as a meadow mushroom.

OTHER TOOLS OF THE TRADE. Over the years, I have seen or heard of many unusual tools that were used to gather mushrooms, including saws, pruning shears, scissors, ladders, and long poles. In his book *Mushrooms of the Great Smokies*, L. R. Hesler recommends snipping the small caps of thick clumps of edible inky caps with scissors instead of picking the caps laboriously by hand. Other mushroomers suggest using saws to cut off a section of a log containing succulent fungi. The log section can be brought home and placed in a garden to produce "home-grown" mushrooms. Ladders and poles are also included in the repertoire of tools used to reach mushrooms high up the bole of a tree. In *Wisconsin Mushrooms*, the authors advise, "A fish pole with a loop of stout wire or a knife fastened to its tip is often needed to bring it [an edible mushroom] to earth." Although such gear is not recommended as part of your equipment, it is interesting to see the lengths to which dedicated collectors will go in the pursuit of edible wild mushrooms.

Your First Collecting Trip

After obtaining the correct mushroom equipment, you are now ready to go on your first foray. The season is right; you know what edible mushrooms to expect in that season by reading the appropriate section in Part II of this book, "Through the Year with Mushrooms." You also know that the weather is a key factor in the success of your mushrooming. If the weather has been too dry, very few mushrooms will appear. However, good, soaking rains will yield a prolific number of mushrooms. The smaller mushrooms will spring up first; the larger mushrooms, which need more time to develop, will mature later.

In the woods, you spy what you think is an edible mushroom. To identify this mushroom, you select the photo in this book that illustrates that mushroom; then you study the key characteristics of the mushroom that accompany the drawing in the section describing the mushroom. Are all the characteristics present? What are they? Could this mushroom be confused with any other? If so, note the differences shown in the drawing. Why was this similar mushroom ruled out in your identification?

As you study your mushroom, try to answer such questions as: What is the shape of the cap? What is its color, size, texture? Does the cap have gills? Pores? How long is the stem? Color? Does it have a ring? Where was the mushroom found—on a log or ground? Under birch or oaks? Near a stream? When?

It is important that you sharpen your powers of observation

so that when you see a mushroom, you will automatically note such characteristics. Write this information on a small piece of paper to keep with your mushrooms or put it in a notebook. Your notes should agree with the description of the species given in this book. Once you get in the habit of noting the characteristics of a mushroom for the first time, you will be surprised at how much easier it will be to identify the mushroom the next time.

When collecting edible mushrooms, select only firm specimens. Avoid mushrooms that are limp, old, or bruised. If you find mushrooms that are riddled with holes, discard them. They are probably filled with insect larvae. When these mushrooms are cut open, trails of the larvae, as well as the culprits themselves, may be seen. Some collectors simply cut out the insect-ridden part and save the rest for the pot.

To simplify cleaning of edible mushrooms, remove any dirt, needles, or pieces of wood before you put your mushrooms into the basket. If the stem of a mushroom is saved as well as the cap, cut off the dirt-laden base. This cleaning in the field will relieve you of extra work at home.

Joining Other Collectors

A pleasant way to help you to learn to identify a large number of edible mushrooms is to join a local mycological club. These clubs are located in various parts of the country, and are composed of amateur mushroom collectors with wide-ranging interests. Although a few members may be interested primarily in identifying or collecting mushrooms, most club members are interested in the culinary possibilities as well. Local clubs usually hold monthly meetings during the winter months and conduct regular field trips during the mushroom season. In each club there are generally several knowledgeable members, perhaps including professional scientists. During a field trip these people can provide a quick mini-course on the identification of edible mushrooms.

For a beginner, the noon break is one of the highlights of the trip. At that time the mushrooms that have been collected are spread out on the ground or on a picnic table. Labels are placed next to the more easily identified mushrooms as one or more of the club's experts explains why a mushroom was identified in a certain way. The more tricky mushrooms trigger a lively discussion and much thumbing through the pages of esoteric guidebooks. If the novice has a question, someone will gladly provide the answer.

A local mushroom club may also conduct a weekend foray or band together with other mycological groups in a region. In the Northeast, for example, mycological groups from Connecticut, Massachusetts, New York, New Hampshire, and New Jersey hold one large regional foray a year. An ambitious program is planned, and an outstanding mushrooming area is chosen with facilities to house as many as 200 persons. Starting on Friday night and lasting to Sunday afternoon, the foray's program would include a variety of walks; talks on mushroom identification, toxicity, and edibility; and sample mushroom tastings. Scientific experts present talks and act as official foray mycologists. Such a weekend is another invaluable way to become quickly exposed to a wide range of mushrooms.

Perhaps the World Series of the weekend mushroom forays is the one held annually by the North American Mycological Association (NAMA), the national organization of amateur mycological groups. Long weekend forays have been held in the Rocky Mountains, in the hills of North Carolina, at Dartmouth College in New Hampshire, in the midwestern state of Ohio, and in the San Francisco region, to name a few locations. A beginner attending one of these forays can view and study at leisure hundreds of mushrooms neatly grouped and labeled and placed on rows of tables.

In addition to organizing the national foray, NAMA also publishes a newsletter and a scientific journal, McIlvainea, named after Charles McIlvaine, the pioneering amateur mycologist of the early twentieth century. Membership is open to anyone interested in learning more about mushrooms. For information, write to North American Mycological Assocation, 4245 Redinger Road, Portsmouth, Ohio, 45662. A list of all the amateur organizations in the United States and Canada appears at the end of this book. Contact any of these groups for local membership information.

A professional organization of mycologists, the Mycological Society of America, is also open to persons interested in mushrooms. Research and industrial scientists and college and university professors make up most of the membership. The organization publishes the technical scientific journal, *Mycologia* (address: New York Botanical Garden, Bronx, New York 10458). Although articles of interest to mycophagists (persons who enjoy eating edible mushrooms) occasionally appear in the journal, only those who have been studying mushrooms for years and are strongly interested in the more technical aspects of fungi would benefit by joining this organization.

Part II

Through the Year with Mushrooms

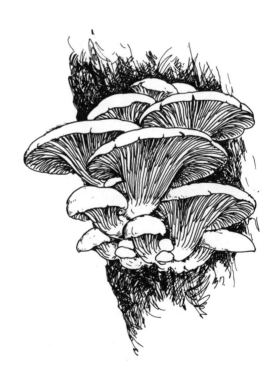

Spring

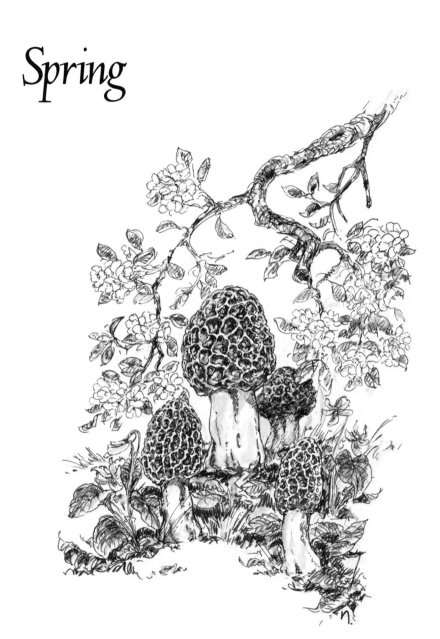

As the silvery buds of the pussy willows emerge and the spring peepers voice their approval of the end of winter, mushroom hunters get ready for another year of collecting. The warm weather and rains of spring trigger a large fruiting of mushrooms. Morels, false morels, colorful cup fungi—thin brittle disk or cup-shaped mushrooms that daub the ground with red, orange, or brown—and a number of gilled mushrooms make their appearance. Although there may not be the wide range of edible species that is found in late summer and fall, the spring season more than makes up for this deficiency by providing perhaps the most delicious of all fungi—the morels.

The early bird of the morels is the black morel (*Morchella angusticeps*). Its dark brown to black spongy head appears in the woodlands when the bracken ferns are still furled in their fiddleheads, when the hepatica, trailing arbutus, and white violets bloom along the woodland trails, and when the first asparagus spears thrust up near the rhubarb in the garden. Although the black morel is the first of the true morels (*Morchella*) to appear, many people have already been collecting what they call an "early morel" (*Verpa bohemica*), which is really a false morel.

Next in the morel spring parade is the common morel (*Morchella esculenta*); it appears in apple orchards, woodlands, around old elms, and near gardens. The seasoned morel hunter looks for the mushroom when apple trees are just beginning to acquire a white coat of blossoms and oak leaves are as big as a squirrel's ear. Next comes the thick-footed morel (*Morchella crassipes*), a fungus that may grow up to a foot tall. This mushroom is found in woodlands, in open places, at the edge of the woods, and in rich garden soil. And finally, ending the morel season, is the tiny white morel (*Morchella deliciosa*), an inhabitant of low, moist woodlands.

For the beginner, the white morel marks the end of the spring collecting season. Although the more experienced collector will also pick other edible mushrooms, the beginner, to avoid possible confusion with nonedible species, will limit the gathering to the several spring morels.

With the morels, you couldn't ask for a better introduction to the world of edible mushrooms.

Morel
(Morchella)

COMMON MOREL (*Morchella esculenta*)
THICK-FOOTED MOREL (*Morchella crassipes*)
BLACK MOREL (*Morchella angusticeps*)
WHITE MOREL (*Morchella deliciosa*)

The morels are perhaps the easiest group of mushrooms to recognize. Morels have a spongelike crown perched on a pale, hollow stem (see Color Plates 1–3). This spongy cap is attached directly to the brittle white to yellowish stem at the base of the crown; both cap and stem are hollow. If the morel is cut in half (Figure 4), the hollow interior is readily visible. Once a beginner has seen a photograph of a true morel, it is almost impossible to confuse it with any other mushroom.

In his book *Common Edible Mushrooms*, Clyde M. Christensen listed the morel as one of the "foolproof four" among wild mushrooms. These mushrooms, says Dr. Christensen, "are considered to be four of the most easily and surely recognized, most abundant and widespread, and most desirable in flavor and texture of all our common edible mushrooms." The other mushrooms placed by Christensen in this category are shaggy manes, puffballs, and sulfur shelf mushrooms.

The most famous and widely distributed morel is the common morel, *Morchella esculenta* (Color Plate 1), This mushroom, which the French call *morille*, is generally 2 to 5 inches high and has a yellow-brown to brown spongy head. The stem is white or yellowish. The inside of the mushroom is entirely hollow. *Mor-*

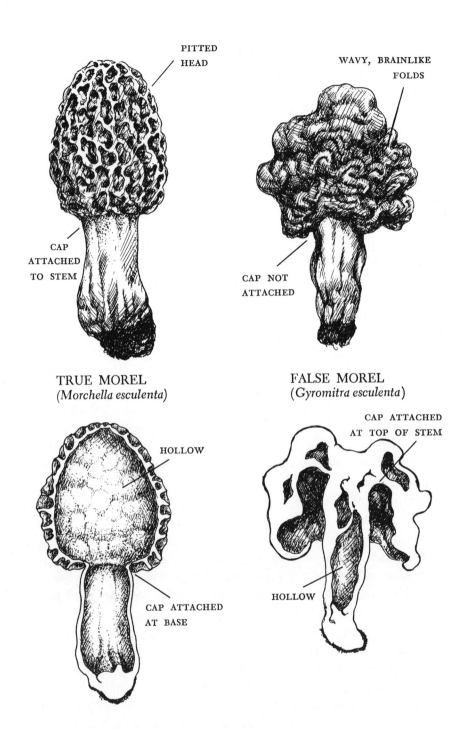

PITTED HEAD

WAVY, BRAINLIKE FOLDS

CAP ATTACHED TO STEM

CAP NOT ATTACHED

TRUE MOREL
(Morchella esculenta)

FALSE MOREL
(Gyromitra esculenta)

HOLLOW

CAP ATTACHED AT TOP OF STEM

CAP ATTACHED AT BASE

HOLLOW

FIGURE 4. *Key features of the true morel and the look-alike false morel.*

chella esculenta is found in a wide variety of habitats. Apple orchards where the soil hasn't been disturbed for many years is one favorite place. Other popular growing areas include open woodlands, evergreen forests, along fence rows, and low, wet areas. The common morel grows in so many different locations that mycologists no longer think that morels form a special mycorrhizal relationship with certain trees, as many other mushrooms do.

One of the tragedies of the American scene, the demise of the stately elm tree due to a fungus disease, has ironically triggered the growth of the common morel in the Midwest, East, and other areas where the elm is found. For some reason, just after an elm tree dies, morels begin sprouting around the base of the tree. The morels don't show up when the tree is dying, nor do they appear too many years after the tree's death. They simply proliferate just after the tree dies and for several years after that. In Ohio and other states, mycologists report brief, large fruitings around elms each spring for several years. Then, the morels are never seen again.

In Massachusetts, where the common morel is not as common in woodlands as in other regions of the United States, one collector looks for morels only around dead elms along country roads. Each year, he obtains enough of these delicious morels to supply a nearby French restaurant and himself with many meals. Why fruiting conditions are ideal just after an elm dies is still a mystery.

The "Bigfoot" of the morel group is the thick-footed morel (*Morchella crassipes*). The Latin name for the mushroom, *crassipes*, means "thick foot." The large, tan, spongy mushroom has a stem with a wide, sometimes grooved footlike base. The mushroom sometimes achieves a height of 1 foot, which is large for a morel. The usually elongated cap has large, shallow pits with thin ridges. The valleys or inside of the pits are yellowish. The thick-footed morel is found in habitats similar to those of the common morel.

Although the thick-footed morel is still generally considered as a separate species, some mycologists have concluded that this fungus is simply a larger variety of the common morel. In one experiment, scientists tagged mushrooms that seemed to be common morels. Upon returning to the site two weeks later, the scientists

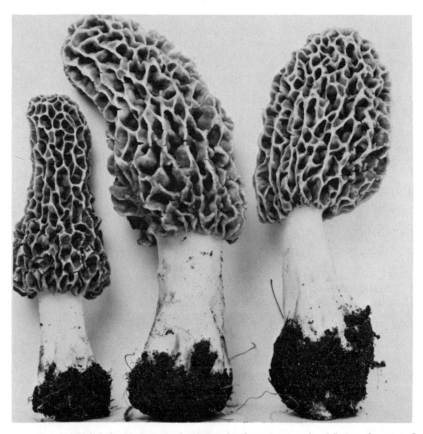

FIGURE 5. *Thick-footed morel* (Morchella crassipes). *Note elongated cap on the two mushrooms on the left.*

discovered that the tagged mushrooms had grown into thick-footed morels. When young, the two species appear indistinguishable. As the thick-footed morel grows older, it becomes much larger than the common morel; the spongy head grows longer (Figure 5), and the foot also becomes more prominent. Because of its large size and delicious taste, the thick-footed morel is widely sought.

The size of this mushroom has spawned some tall stories. Commercial fishermen in Michigan tell of harvesting foot-high morels from their boats, and claim that the morels, which grow at the shores of islands, are so numerous that they look like big blobs of foam that have been washed ashore.

Another abundant morel is *Morchella angusticeps*, the black morel. Like the common morel, the black morel is found throughout the United States. The black morel is slender, 2 to 5 inches tall, and when fully grown has a dark, spongelike head. The pits on the head are long and narrow and are stacked one above the other in vertical rows. The stem is cream to buff colored. When the mushroom first thrusts up through the soil, its cap is pale tan or gray-brown. As it becomes older, the ridges on the cap turn almost black (Color Plate 2). Hence, the name black morel. The dark cap looks like a slender upside-down ice cream cone.

The black morel may be found on sandy soil in the woods and at the border of woodlands where oak, aspen, and other trees grow. The black morel is a common inhabitant of evergreen forests. Perhaps one of the mushroom's most interesting preferences is for areas that have just been burned. Each spring in the West, experienced morel collectors congregate in any area that was swept by forest fire the previous year. The black morels, looking like charred remnants of the fire, spring up by the bushel in the burn. Although *Morchella esculenta* may also be found in the burned area, the black morels are by far the most abundant. This prolific fruiting is best the first year after the fire, less so the second year, perhaps nonexistent the next. Apparently, the ashes provide these morels with the right mix of nutrients for proliferation.

A morel's affinity for scorched areas has been recognized for many centuries. In the Middle Ages, German peasants would deliberately burn the woodland understory to encourage the growth of these succulent mushrooms. The practice became so commonplace that officials passed a law in the eighteenth century forbidding such acts. In the United States, this practice exists, but on a much smaller scale, among midwestern farmers who burn the grassy undergrowth of large apple orchards to spur the growth of morels.

In the Pacific Northwest and in some other regions of the United States, there is another dark morel that grows much taller and broader than the narrow-capped *Morchella angusticeps*. Unlike the typical *Morchella angusticeps*, this large morel has a blackish cap from the time the mushroom emerges from the ground until it dies. The mushroom grows up to 7 inches tall and has a broad conical cap 3 to 4 inches in diameter; it begins to appear about a week later than the common *Morchella angusticeps*. The mushroom is considered a large variety of the smaller, more narrow-capped black morel (*Morchella angusticeps*). The mushroom is widely collected and delicious eating, although some cases of illness (gastrointestinal upsets) have been reported in the Pacific Northwest among people eating this mushroom. Perhaps specimens that were too old were eaten in these cases. Only young, fresh specimens should be collected. Discard any mushrooms that have begun to deteriorate. Even among *Morchella angusticeps*, mushrooms that have a completely blackened head and have begun to shrink should not be collected; they are past their prime.

Although the white morel (*Morchella deliciosa*) trails the black morel and other morels in seasonal appearance, the Latin name for this morel shows that it compares favorably in taste. The white morel is a very small mushroom, only 1½ to 3 inches tall. It is found in grassy areas, usually at the edge of woodlands. Low, moist forests containing ash, elm, and red maple are good areas for collectors. Although the mushroom is widely distributed in the United States, it is not as abundant as the common morel. The white morel is named for the white to pallid ridges that contrast sharply with the deep brown pits and the white stem that is often enlarged at the base (Color Plate 3).

When collecting morels for the table, the beginner should avoid confusing the true morels with a group of mushrooms known as the false morels. Although several species of false morels have been collected and eaten without harm for many years, poisonings have occurred. False morels may contain toxins known as gyromitrin and monomethylhydrazine (see p. 25). Although many collectors claim that toxins can be removed from the mushrooms by parboiling them and then throwing away the water, this method does not always work. It is best to avoid problems by not eating false morels.

The true morels can be readily distinguished from the false morels, although the species may seem similar at first glance. (See Figure 4 and Color Plates 1–5.) Figure 4 illustrates the key differences between a true morel (*Morchella esculenta*) and a typical false morel (*Gyromitra esculenta*). A true morel, as mentioned earlier, has a spongy cap or head with deep pits and ridges. The false morels have a cap that is either nearly smooth, wrinkled, or folded like the folds of a brain. The cap is often shaped like a saddle. *The cap is never pitted.* Another key difference is that the base of the cap of the true morel is connected directly to the stalk. In the false morels, the cap or head hangs like a skirt, away from the stem, and is attached only at the top of the stem.

The false morels may be divided into three main groups (*Gyromitra, Helvella,* and *Verpa*). *Gyromitra* means "round miter," *Helvella,* a "small pot herb," and *Verpa,* a "rod." Although there are various technical differences between *Gyromitra* and *Helvella,* a general rule in the field is that the *Helvella* species are white, pale gray to black, while the *Gyromitras* are yellow, tan, to red-brown. The variation of the color on *Gyromitra esculenta* can be readily seen in Color Plate 4.

Species of *Verpa,* the third group of mushrooms that are frequently lumped with false morels, can also be easily distinguished from the true morels. The key distinction is that the *Verpa* cap is attached only at the top of the stem, so that the caps form the typical skirt of a false morel. *Verpa* caps are also smooth to wrinkled. In one species, *Verpa bohemica,* the skirtlike cap may vary from wrinkled folds to long ridges that may at times resemble long pits; but, again, the attachment to the top of the stem gives the mushroom away. The range in folding in the skirtlike cap of this species is shown in Color Plate 5. *Verpa bohemica* is popularly called the "early morel" even though it is not a true morel. "So many people eat and enjoy this species that it cannot fairly be labelled poisonous," says Alexander Smith in the *Mushroom Hunter's Field Guide.* However, when eaten in large amounts, this mushroom can cause lack of muscular coordination and stomach upsets, making it one of those species that is reportedly poisonous for some people but not for others. To avoid any problems, beginners should stay only with the true morels.

Another species of mushroom is sometimes grouped with the true morels and sometimes with the false morels. This edible mushroom, popularly called the cow's head, half-free morel, or the hybrid morel, combines the characteristics of a true morel and a *Verpa.* It has a cap that is sometimes pitted like a morel or wrin-

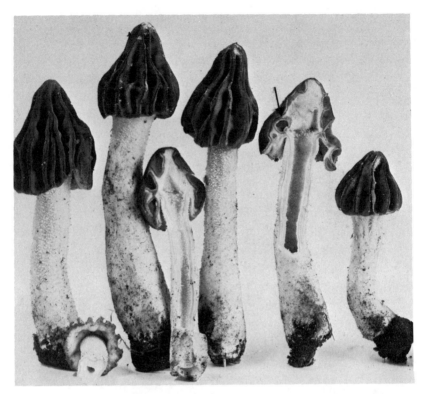

FIGURE 6. *Half-free morel* (Morchella semilibera). *Note how the cap attaches part way up the stalk in the mushroom that has been cut into two sections. A small hollow area (arrow) can be seen in each section above the point of attachment.*

kled to ridged like a *Verpa bohemica*; however, the cap, instead of connecting at the apex of the stem as in the false morels, is attached halfway up the stalk (Figure 6). With a "miniskirt" cap that is sometimes pitted, this species seems to straddle the line between a true morel and a false morel. Some mycologists place this species with the morels and call it *Morchella semilibera*; others categorize it as a separate genus. Alexander Smith thinks it may belong with the *Verpas*, because in very young fruiting bodies of this mushroom, the head is at first attached to the apex of the stalk. As the cap grows longer, a hollow area develops between the apex and the original point of attachment. Because of this hollow, the cap at maturity *appears* to be attached about midway up the stalk. If, in fact, this mushroom does end up with *Verpas*, it will be the one exception to the rule that false morels are never pitted. Even though this species is edible, the beginner should stay with the common morel, the thick-footed morel, the black morel, and the delicious morel.

Morels may appear as early as February in the Deep South of the United States and in April or May farther north. Morel collectors in each region will use the seasonal clues mentioned earlier to determine when to start looking for particular species. The growing season for each species is brief, usually only a few weeks. In particular regions, such as the Midwest, morels are so abundant that bushels of them can easily be collected in a day in a relatively small area. In some rural areas, students may skip school to collect morels in the woods, appearing later along the roadside with bags of morels to sell.

Morels are most abundant during a wet spring; however, their appearance from year to year in specific areas isn't always predictable. Sometimes morels will appear in the same spot on the same hillside for several years in a row. Or they will fruit in great numbers in one area during one year and then disappear from that spot for several years. The proper mix of temperature and the amount of moisture needed for fruiting is known only to the morel.

Morels blend with their surroundings. Their muted colors provide such excellent camouflage in the leafy duff that you could easily pass a clump of these mushrooms without seeing them. But if you are alert, one morel may suddenly materialize. Then its neighbors will also be seen standing out in a Lilliputian forest. Although mushroom collectors are normally friendly, the quickest way to strain a mycophile's friendship is to ask where he or she finds morels. It's like asking a fisherman where his favorite fishing hole is. Your question may elicit a polite refusal, a deft switch to another subject, or an uncomfortable silence caused by the listener's sudden attack of "morelitis," a disease whose main symptom is temporary deafness.

The devotion of morel buffs to their craft is legendary. Some like to tell the story of a soldier, James Nathan Miller, who was attached to an American Division during its sweep through Germany in the last stages of World War II. Just as his division was about to make its historic linkup with the Russian troops east of Leipzig, Miller discovered some morels in the woodlands. War or no war, Miller promptly prepared a handful of freshly picked morels which he consumed with a bottle of German wine.

Perhaps the lure of the morel reaches its zenith each spring in Boyne City, a small ski-resort town in northern Michigan. Each second weekend in May, the town, which bills itself as the Morel Mushroom Capital of the World, holds a National Mushroom Picking Contest. One purpose of the contest is to see how many morels a contestant can pick in ninety minutes. At the crack of a starting gun, contestants of all ages and from as far away as Kentucky, spring from the starting line and head for the woods. At this time of year, the woodlands are usually liberally sprinkled with several species of morels. The contest favors the fleet of foot and the collector with a practiced eye. A sensitive nose for smelling the morels also helps, one winner from Ohio insists.

After ninety minutes, the contestants bring their bounty to the collecting point to be tallied. On Sunday evening, a dinner is held at the local Masonic Lodge where the winners as well as the losers share the morels. For those interested in records, Stan Boris of Boyne City holds the record for collecting the greatest number of morels. In 1971, Stan tallied 915 morels in 90 minutes, a rate of about 10 morels a minute.

The brief collecting season for the morel causes morel enthusiasts to yearn for *fresh* morels the year round. Fortunately, morels preserve very well by drying; yet morelists wish that researchers could develop a method for growing morels commercially. Spurring them on are accounts in early French garden and scientific journals describing how morels were grown in flowerpots and in gardens. In experiments in the early part of the twentieth century, morels were grown successfully in beds of artichokes and in beds containing a residue of apples and paper waste—an unusual combination. In these experiments, spawn grown by the scientists was used to start the growth of morels. In one study, nearly a pound of morels was obtained for every square yard planted. There is no problem in growing morels from spawn, says Rolf Singer in *Mushrooms and Truffles*. The problem occurs when scientists try to adapt the results of these small-scale experiments to the large-scale production of commercial morels.

In the United States, when an attempt was made to cultivate morels commercially, a large growth of mycelia was obtained, but no morel fruiting. One company then produced a powder from the mycelia. The powder, which is no longer available, was used as a seasoning in soups and gravies. Although the powder supposedly had a good flavor, purists, who feel that seeing the morel nuggets is part of the total dining experience, would not be satisfied.

With regard to wild morels, a few rules of caution must be observed. Don't eat them raw. Raw morels have given some people upset stomachs. Unless stated otherwise in this book for a particular species, eat only cooked mushrooms. Morels should not be consumed with alcohol, James Nathan Miller notwithstanding, because some cases of stomach upsets have been recently recorded as a result of this combination.

What is it about morels that elevates this mushroom to such high favor? Sauté one morel in butter or margarine and then sample it and you will find the answer. The aroma that fills your kitchen during the sautéing will remind you of the damp leafy places from whence the mushroom came. The mushroom has a woodsy flavor that is superb and worthy of all the praise that it has received over the centuries.

When preparing these mushrooms, the flavor should, as with all fine foods, be enhanced, not masked. Do not overwhelm the morels with seasonings and other foods. Morels are delicious simply sautéed, added to eggs, stuffed, or in a cream sauce that will accompany beef or fish.

NOTE: The number accompanying each of the following mushroom descriptions refers to that mushroom's color plate in the color insert. The edibility designation of each mushroom is based on the following edibility scale:

Edible—ranges from good to very good to delicious (the highest rating).

Inedible—not poisonous, but not good to eat because of undesirable qualities such as bitterness.

Poisonous—the mushroom has an adverse effect, which may range from a mild to severe poisoning. Mushrooms that may affect only some collectors are also included. When the word *deadly* is added after the word *poisonous*, it's self-explanatory. You will find the white amanita, the destroying angel, described as "deadly."

1 Common Morel   EDIBLE, DELICIOUS

Morchella esculenta
("mushroom" "edible")

COMMON NAMES

Sponge mushroom, pine cone fungus, the morel, honeycomb, corn cob, common morel, merkle, myrtles, Molly moocher, mountain fish, yellow morel.

WHAT IT LOOKS LIKE

Cap: 2 to 4 inches long, deeply pitted like a sponge or weather-beaten honeycomb; oval to almost cone shaped, yellow-brown to other shades of brown; ridges typically lighter than pits; hollow. *Stem:* ½ to 4 inches tall, fragile, white to cream; inside of stalk feels as if coated with bumpy white kid leather; slightly enlarged at base, sometimes wrinkled, hollow. *Spores:* yellowish.

KEY FEATURES

Brown, spongelike head; hollow interior and cap connected to the stem at base of cap.

WHERE FOUND

Widely distributed throughout North America. In old apple orchards, under elms, in low, wet areas, lightly burned grassy areas, woodlands. Occurs singly or in small groups. Abundant during wet spring.

WHEN

When apple trees and lilacs are in blossom and the oak leaves are about the size of squirrel ears. Usually in May in northern part of the United States, earlier farther south.

2 Black Morel   EDIBLE, DELICIOUS
Morchella angusticeps
("mushroom" "narrow head")

COMMON NAMES

Black morel, narrow-capped morel, mountain fish, slender-capped morel.

WHAT IT LOOKS LIKE

Cap: ¾ to 2½ inches long, narrow pitted head; resembles a slender upside-down cone; pits are dull brown and long, ridges turn from pale tan or gray-brown to almost black with age; ridges between long pits form distinct vertical lines bridged by cross ridges; hollow. *Stem:* ¾ to 2½ inches tall, flaky, hollow, nearly as thick as the head; cream to buff colored. *Spores:* yellowish.

KEY FEATURES

Dark brown-black ridges on a narrow, spongy, hollow cap attached at base to a hollow stem.

WHERE FOUND

In evergreen regions of North America, in apple orchards, along roadsides, in aspen stands, and in oak and other hardwood forests. Fruits in great numbers in areas where a forest fire has occurred. A large black variety is also found, particularly in the Pacific Northwest.

WHEN

Fruits early in the spring when the fiddleheads appear, when the first asparagus spears pierce the surface, when the hepatica and violets bloom, and before the aspen leaves are out. First of the true morels described here to appear.

3 White Morel   EDIBLE, DELICIOUS
Morchella deliciosa
("mushroom" "delicious")

COMMON NAMES
White morel, delicious morel.

WHAT IT LOOKS LIKE
Cap: ¾ to 1½ inches long; looks like honeycomb, ridges are whitish, pits deep brown; hollow. *Stem:* ¾ to 1½ inches tall; pale, hollow, and often wider at the base. *Spores:* yellowish.

KEY FEATURES
Spongy hollow cap with white ridges and brown pits; cap is attached to hollow stem at its base.

WHERE FOUND
In grassy areas, usually at edge of woods. In low, moist forests. Widely distributed, but not common.

WHEN
One of the last morels to appear in spring.

4 False Morel   POISONOUS
Gyromitra esculenta
("round miter"   "edible")

COMMON NAMES
Brain mushroom, false morel, lorchel, elephant ear, beefsteak morel.

WHAT IT LOOKS LIKE
Cap: 1 to 4 inches across; wavy, wrinkled folds like the lobes of a brain, NOT PITTED; yellowish brown to dark reddish brown;

smooth when young; cap attached at top of stem. *Stem:* ¾ to 2 inches tall; white or brownish; hollow, sometimes compressed or pinched into two hollows. *Spores:* yellowish.

KEY FEATURES

The wrinkled, brainlike folds, absence of pitting, and the cap attached at the top of the stem distinguish this false morel from true morels.

WHERE FOUND

Evergreen forests seem to be the favorite habitat of the false morel or brain mushroom.

WHEN

Early spring and on into June or early summer in the more mountainous areas of the United States.

5 Early Morel   POISONOUS
Verpa bohemica
("rod" "Bohemia")

COMMON NAMES

Early morel, false morel.

WHAT IT LOOKS LIKE

Cap: ¾ to 1¼ inches long; bell- or thimble-shaped, hangs free from stem, attached only at top of stem; wrinkled up and down the cap, yellow-brown. *Stem:* 1¼ to 3¼ inches tall; cream colored; hollow or partly filled with "cottony" material. *Spores:* yellowish.

KEY FEATURES

Small, skirt-like cap attached at top of stem; cap has surface that varies from wrinkled folds to long "pits."

WHERE FOUND

Likes rich soil in low, wet areas such as along edges of swamps, and along riverbanks. In the West, the mushroom prefers stream valleys under cottonwood, willows, and aspens.

WHEN

Appears in early spring, before the leaves appear on the trees.

Summer

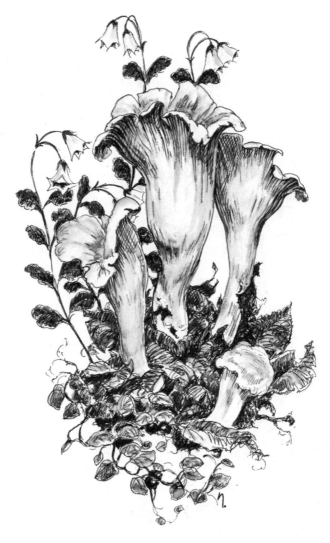

In the world of fungi, the early part of summer means bright color. The warm summer rains of July bring out the first russulas as well as the milky lactarius mushrooms. These stocky mushrooms with the wide-brimmed caps paint the woodland floor with bright reds and oranges, contrasting sharply with a few early white coral fungi. The deadly white amanitas also appear, like wood-land ghosts, next to the colorful russulas or lactarius fungi.

My favorite bright early-summer mushroom is the trumpet-shaped golden chanterelle (*Cantharellus cibarius*). This delicious yellow mushroom with the vaulted ribs along its sides grows in large groups beneath evergreen canopies. Two other closely re-lated edible mushrooms, the gill-less chanterelle (*Craterellus cantharellus*) and the dark horn of plenty (*Craterellus cornucopio-ides*), may also be found at this time.

As the summer progresses, another summer edible, the beau-tiful sulphur shelf mushroom (*Polyporus sulphureus*), graces logs, trees, and stumps with shelves of orange and yellow caps. Summer boletes and polypores proliferate after rains. In August, a cool spell with showers will trigger the fruiting of meadow mushrooms (*Agaricus campestris*) as they form fairy rings on lawns and meadows. Puffballs (*Calvatia*) dot the grounds like loaves of bread.

In the woodlands, some unusual edible mushrooms with "teeth" or "icicles" also appear. They drape in iciclelike white clusters (*Hericium*) from logs or stumps, while other toothed fungi with cap and stem (*Dentinum repandum* and *Dentinum umbilicatum*) grow in low, moist soil along woodland streams or bogs. In the mountains of the West, relatives of the lowland puff-balls can be found in the warted giant puffballs of the high ever-green forests (*Calbovista subsculpta*). More gilled mushrooms, such as the *Clitocybes*, spring up out of the ground. When the hot weather returns again in August, the outburst of mushrooms triggered by the month's rains will wane. And it will be time to look ahead to the "big season," the fall of the year—at least in terms of numbers of fruiting.

Vase-shaped Mushroom

(*Cantharellus* and *Craterellus*)

GOLDEN CHANTERELLE (*Cantharellus cibarius*)
WHITE CHANTERELLE (*Cantharellus subalbidus*)
GILL-LESS CHANTERELLE (*Craterellus cantharellus*)
HORN OF PLENTY (*Craterellus cornucopioides*)

In Germany, it is called the *pfifferling*; in Scandinavia, the *kantarellas*; in France, the *girolle* or *chanterelle*. On the continent of Europe alone, more than two hundred local or regional names have been appended to this vase-shaped mushroom—a true testament to its popularity. The mushroom (Figure 7) is the golden chanterelle (*Cantharellus cibarius*). The chanterelle has long been a favorite of Europeans. Each summer, people from the coast of France eastward to Russia, and from Scandinavia south to the boot of Italy swarm into the open woodlands to collect these mushrooms that look like daubs of gold in the rich woodland soil. The mushrooms are sometimes so plentiful that hundreds will carpet the woodland floor over a small area. Many are collected and sold in public markets. R. W. and F. W. Rolfe, in *The Romance of the Fungus World*, note that of the approximately 26,000 pounds of wild mushrooms that were sold during one season in the city of Lyons, France, the golden chanterelle was by far the most popular wild mushroom.

This egg-yellow mushroom with ribbed arches looks like a diminutive vaulted column from a Gothic cathedral. Blunt ridges

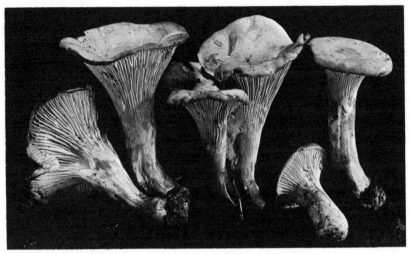

FIGURE 7. *Golden chanterelle* (Cantharellus cibarius).

or ribs along the outside arch seem to support the cap. Smaller interconnecting bridges between the ribs add still more solidity. Actually, the outside surface containing the ribbed superstructure has a more mundane function. The spores are produced there.

Scientists include the golden chanterelle in the genus *Cantharellus*. The name is derived from a Greek word meaning "vase" or "cup." This group of mushrooms typically has a vaselike or trumpet-shaped fruiting body with blunt edges rather than knife-like gills on the outside or underside of the cap (Figure 8 and Color Plate 6B). These blunt edges travel down the cap and merge with the stipe.

The golden chanterelle is a cosmopolitan mushroom, growing in temperate regions in such disparate countries as India and Japan, as well as in Europe and the United States. The golden chanterelle is not a large mushroom (Color Plate 6A). The cap is generally about 1 to 3 inches across, and the mushroom grows to about the same height. Its flesh is thick and meaty. In Europe the mushroom always has a fragrant, fruity odor of apricots; however, the fruity odor is sometimes not noticeable in the U.S. chanterelle.

Although many species of chanterelles grow in various regions of the United States, a beginner should focus only on four closely related and easily recognized vase- or trumpet-shaped mushrooms. They are the egg-yellow golden chanterelle (*Cantharellus cibarius*), which is widely distributed throughout the country; the white chanterelle (*Cantharellus subalbidus*), a species of the Pacific Northwest often found growing with the golden chanterelle; the gill-less yellowish chanterelle (*Craterellus cantharellus*) an eastern species; and the dark horn of plenty (*Craterellus cornucopioides*), a delicious mushroom that is often used in recipes as a substitute for truffles. The spore-bearing surface of the latter two mushrooms, the outside of the vase, is very smooth to barely wrinkled, whereas in the golden and white chanterelles, the blunt gill edges are more prominent. This characteristic places the gill-less chanterelle and the horn of plenty mushrooms in the closely related genus, *Craterellus*. All four of these species are distinctive enough so that by following the guidelines in this section you should not confuse them with any other species. As you become more knowledgeable, you can graduate to other edible chanterelles and more comprehensive mushroom books that identify all of these fungi.

The golden chanterelle generally begins appearing in midsummer after a rain. It continues to fruit throughout the summer and into early fall. A good, wet summer will cause these colorful fungi to proliferate. Rich woodland soil is the favorite habitat of the chanterelle; the mushroom grows in both evergreen and deciduous forests. I have found clusters of these egg-yellow fungi in the sylvan shade of hemlock stands, in the most soil along woodland streams, and in the rich humus of open oak woods. The mushrooms may be scattered throughout the woodland duff, form curved lines, or cluster in large groups sometimes numbering in the hundreds. A group of amateur mycologists on a foray may sometimes collect as much as 20 pounds of chanterelles in a small area. If a similar amount of canned chanterelles imported from Europe were purchased in a store, these mushrooms would cost about $320. (A small can of European chanterelles containing approximately 8 ounces of mushrooms sells for about $8).

Two species of mushrooms can be confused with the golden chanterelle. One, the beautiful jack-o'-lantern fungus (*Omphalotus illudens*) is poisonous. It can cause stomach upsets and diarrhea. The second, the false chanterelle (*Hygrophoropsis aurantiacus*), although widely eaten in Europe without ill effect and touted by some authorities in this country as edible, may cause illness in

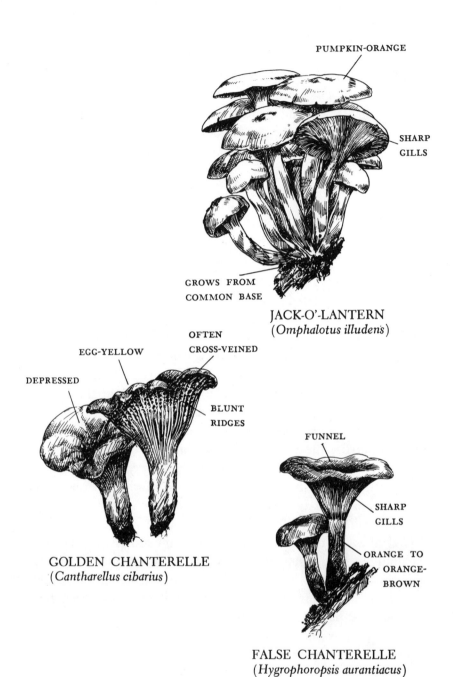

PUMPKIN-ORANGE

SHARP
GILLS

GROWS FROM
COMMON BASE

JACK-O'-LANTERN
(*Omphalotus illudens*)

OFTEN
CROSS-VEINED

EGG-YELLOW

DEPRESSED

BLUNT
RIDGES

FUNNEL

SHARP
GILLS

ORANGE TO
ORANGE-
BROWN

GOLDEN CHANTERELLE
(*Cantharellus cibarius*)

FALSE CHANTERELLE
(*Hygrophoropsis aurantiacus*)

FIGURE 8. *Key features of the golden chanterelle* (Cantharellus cibarius) *and two look-alikes.*

some people. However, by carefully observing a few simple rules, the golden chanterelle (*Cantharellus cibarius*) can be easily distinguished from these two mushrooms (Figure 8).

The golden chanterelle is egg-yellow, has blunt or dull-edged forked gills that are often bridged by cross veins, and grows in scattered groups on the ground.

The jack-o'-lantern has a cap the color of a pumpkin, has sharp gills that look like the edges of knife blades, and grows in a dense clump from a common base at the foot of stumps (Color Plate 7). It grows on wood and usually fruits from the underground parts of an old tree or stump. Another important difference—the reason why the jack-o'-lantern received its name—is that the mushroom glows in the dark. The golden chanterelle does not. I have taken a large cluster of a jack-o'-lantern into a dark basement, and within a few minutes the gills began to luminesce, forming a delicate pale-green network of glowing parallel lines. The fungus luminesced each time I brought a collected sample into a dark room. The luminescence may persist for a long time. One mushroom collector was able to read a newspaper by the light given off by a clump of these mushrooms three days after the fungus was collected.

The luminescent test, the growth of the jack-o'-lantern from one source on wood, its orange color, and its sharp gills are all characteristics that should easily separate this mushroom from the golden chanterelle.

The second confusing species, the false chanterelle (*Hygrophoropsis aurantiacus*), may also be ruled out in several ways. The color is one important characteristic: the false chanterelle is orange to orange-brown, not an overall egg-yellow like the golden chanterelle. The distinct orange color has resulted in another common name for this mushroom—the orange chanterelle. The scientific name for this mushroom (*aurantiacus*) also means orange.

The false or orange chanterelle, like the jack-o'-lantern fungus, has knife-edge gills; no cross veins connect the crowded bright orange gills as in the golden chanterelle. Its funnel-shaped cap also looks like an umbrella that has become inverted by fierce winds. The mushroom grows directly on soil or on partially decayed wood in the forest. Many mushroom specialists consider the orange chanterelle edible.

Gary Lincoff, co-author of *Toxic and Hallucinogenic Mushroom Poisoning*, thinks that people who were reportedly poisoned by eating the false or orange chanterelle in the United States may have been eating the jack-o'-lantern fungus, under the assumption that they were eating the orange chanterelle. Until more definite information is available, it is best to stay on the safe side and not eat the mushroom.

All experts concur that the golden chanterelle ranks high on the list of edible mushrooms. It is an extremely versatile mushroom. In addition to its delicious flavor, chanterelles also keep well. They may be dried, stored in the refrigerator for a week before eating, or put into a freezer uncooked or barely sautéed to be used up to a year later. Because the flesh is considerably firmer than that of most other mushrooms, it does not shrink much in cooking. Thus, enough chanterelles can be collected for several meals in a short period of time. The firm chanterelle must be cooked over low heat longer than other mushrooms because of its thick, meaty texture.

The golden chanterelle goes well with many foods. The entire mushroom may be used in cooking. Chanterelles are excellent with scrambled eggs, in sauces, or stewed with meat. They combine naturally with tomatoes or with dishes containing tomato sauce. One of my favorite ways of preparing chanterelles is to sauté them in butter with garlic and parsley and serve them on toast.

In the Pacific Northwest, a short, stocky, white chanterelle (Figure 9) frequently crops up in the woodlands alongside the golden chanterelle. This mushroom (*Cantharellus subalbidus*), with characteristic blunt, often forked, ridges running down the stem, closely resembles *Cantharellus cibarius* except that it is white. The very fleshy mushroom, 2 to 4 inches high, also stains orange-yellow when first bruised, then turns orange-brown. This meaty mushroom grows in evergreen woods and in mixed evergreens in late summer and fall. It is considered one of the best Western edible fungi.

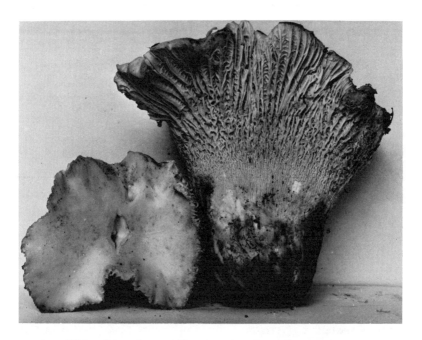

FIGURE 9. *This white chanterelle* (Cantharellus subalbidus) *is found in the same places as the golden chanterelle in the Pacific Northwest. This short, stocky mushroom (1 to 3 inches high) stains orange-yellow when first bruised, then turns to orange-brown. Note the blunt ridges or veins interconnected by smaller bridges of veins in the folds. The white chanterelle has white spores. It grows in groups or in great clusters in the late summer and fall under Douglas fir and other evergreens.*

Another delicious chanterelle vying for top honors in another region is the gill-less chanterelle (*Craterellus cantharellus*). This mushroom is found in the eastern part of the United States, and most frequently in the South and Southeast. The gill-less chanterelle also resembles the golden chanterelle (Color Plate 8). In fact, many people may have eaten it thinking it was *Cantharellus cibarius*. Howard E. Bigelow, in a *Mycologia* article on "The Cantharelloid Fungi of New England and Adjacent Areas," points out that the mushroom may be more common in some areas than originally supposed because of the tendency to confuse this mushroom with the golden chanterelle. Both species are similar in color and shape (see Color Plates 6, 8), but *Craterellus can-*

tharellus has a thinner flesh and its spore-bearing surface is smooth to only slightly wrinkled. In the golden chanterelle the surface is more strongly veined. The difference between the outer surface of the caps can be seen in the color plates of the two species and in the drawing of *Craterellus cantharellus* that introduces the summer section of this book, p. 73. In the drawing, the outer surface of the gill-less chanterelle is smooth. In Color Plate 8, the surface of this chanterelle is not as strongly veined as the veins shown in the color plate (6B) of the golden chanterelle. *Craterellus cantharellus* grows in small to large clusters in hardwood forests in July and August. It is more abundant in wet summers. It is extremely tasty and can be prepared the same way' as the golden chanterelle.

The horn of plenty, which appears in summer and fall at the same time as the golden chanterelle does, is another vase- or trumpet-shaped *Craterellus*. The mushroom (*Craterellus cornucopioides*) looks like a gray to brownish-black trumpet that grows up to 4 inches high (Color Plate 9). The inside of the trumpet is gray-brown, almost like the color of dried leaves. It is completely hollow from the top of the trumpet all the way to the base of the stem. The exterior of the trumpet is smooth to slightly wrinkled, is ash gray, and looks almost frosty. The frosty appearance is due to the spores that coat the surface of the mushroom.

The French call the horn of plenty *trompette du mort* ("trumpet of death"). The name in no way refers to the edible qualities of the mushroom. Instead it was given because of the mushroom's funereal colors and its resemblance to the black trumpets once used in Europe at funerals.

The funnel-shaped horn of plenty may be found in large numbers in woodlands, along old wood roads and trails, among the needles on the floor of evergreen forests, on shaded banks, and among moss and leaf mold. It occurs throughout eastern North America and along the Pacific Coast. While the golden chanterelle cries for attention in the woodlands, the somber gray to brownish-black colors of the horn of plenty among the dead leaves makes it difficult for the casual observer to see. Mushroom collectors can pass by a huge clump of horn of plenty only to have another collector spy the edible fungi. Once one of the mushrooms is spotted, however, the others quickly materialize out of the woodland background. The best way to spot these elusive mushrooms (as well as others) is to stop periodically in a promising area of the woods and look around. You are likely to see mushrooms that would have been missed if you had gone right on.

The mushroom is an excellent-tasting fungus that is worthy of another name by which it is sometimes called: the black truffle. Although not a truffle, French housewives use the horn of plenty in pâtés and other foods as a substitute for truffles. The mushroom has a pleasant aroma when handled, sautéed, or kept in a bag. The thin flesh of the horn of plenty can be easily preserved by drying. When the mushroom is moistened again before reusing, it expands to its normal size. The mushroom can also be preserved by freezing. Like the golden chanterelle, the horn of plenty is delicious with scrambled eggs.

6   Golden Chanterelle   EDIBLE, DELICIOUS

Cantharellus cibarius
("vase"   "food")

COMMON NAMES

Golden chanterelle, yellow chanterelle, egg mushroom, edible chanterelle, pfifferling (and many other regional names brought to the United States by immigrants from Europe).

WHAT IT LOOKS LIKE

Cap: 1 to 3 inches across; slightly dimpled in center, soon becoming shaped like a trumpet or vase, edge of cap wavy or lobed; egg-yolk yellow or paler. *Flesh:* firm, thick, light, yellowish. *Spore-producing Surface:* blunt-edged ridges, not true gills, extend down part of stem (see Color Plate 6B for closeup view of ridges), prominent cross veins often form bridges in depressions between blunt ridges, yellow color of gill-like ridges and stipe sometimes slightly paler than cap. *Stem:* ¾ to 3 inches tall; smooth, solid; yellow, often paler than cap; narrows toward base, thick; may have odor like ripe apricots and a peppery taste (not obvious in many cases). *Spores:* yellowish.

KEY FEATURES

The golden chanterelle has blunt branching ridges or veins, while the two look alikes—the jack-o'-lantern and the false chanterelle—have knife-edged gills. The golden chanterelle is egg yellow, and grows scattered on the ground, while the jack-o'-lantern is pumpkin orange, grows in a clump on wood from a common base, and luminesces. The false chanterelle is orange to orange-brown.

WHERE FOUND

Grows scattered or in groups on the ground in open evergreen and deciduous woods. Widely distributed in forests throughout the United States and Canada.

WHEN

In summer and into fall. In Pacific Northwest, present even late in the fall. In California, fruits late, in winter.

7 Jack-o'-Lantern Fungus   POISONOUS

Omphalotus illudens
"navel"   "deceiving"

COMMON NAMES

Jack-o'-lantern, jack-o'-lantern fungus, false chanterelle.

WHAT IT LOOKS LIKE

Cap: 2 to 4 inches across; flat to slightly curved, often has knob or depression in center, smooth, edge of cap bent down; brilliant pumpkin orange to orange-yellow. *Flesh:* white with tinge of orange; strong, sweet unpleasant odor. *Gills:* like knife blades, spaced close together and very thin; yellow-orange; extend part way down stem; glow in the dark. *Stem:* up to 6 inches tall; often tapers to narrow base; light orange; stalks fuse and form large clump at base; when a stalk is pulled from the clump, it breaks off like a banana from a stem. *Spores:* creamy white.

KEY FEATURES

Bright pumpkin color, knife-edged gills that glow in the dark, and habit of growing in a dense cluster from a common base on wood. Old or dried-out jack-o'-lantern specimens may not luminesce like actively growing jack-o'-lanterns, so one should not rely on this characteristic alone in identifying this mushroom.

WHERE FOUND

Usually occurs in large clumps at the base of old hardwood stumps in eastern North America and across the southern United States to the Pacific Coast. May also grow from buried wood such as a concealed tree root in the ground. Watch for such jack-o'-lanterns that may grow singly in the ground.

WHEN

Late summer and fall.

8 Gill-less Chanterelle

EDIBLE, DELICIOUS

Craterellus cantharellus
("small cup" "vase")

COMMON NAMES

Gill-less chanterelle.

WHAT IT LOOKS LIKE

Cap: 1 to 3½ inches across; rounded, becoming depressed and funnel shaped; edge of cap wavy to ruffled; orange when young, pale yellow when older. *Flesh:* Thin; white, orange near surface; rather brittle. *Spore-producing Surface:* smooth at first, becoming slightly wrinkled with age; orange-yellow to yellow to pinkish from spores. *Stem:* 1 to 3 inches tall; solid, often hollow; tapers toward base, or slightly enlarged at either end; light orange-yellow to color of spore surface, flesh white. *Spores:* light yellow-orange to salmon pink.

KEY FEATURES

The thinner flesh and smooth to slightly wrinkled spore surface of this edible chanterelle provide a sharp contrast with the more strongly veined, more solid golden chanterelle. Largely because of its thinner flesh and hollow stipe, *Cantharellus odoratus* was once considered a separate but closely related species. Now it has been categorized with *Craterellus cantharellus* as one species. Its characteristic hollow stipe has been incorporated into the general description of this mushroom.

WHERE FOUND

Grows in small to large clusters in eastern North America. Although normally considered most abundant in the South and Southeast, it may be more common elsewhere than originally thought.

WHEN

Summer.

9 Horn of Plenty   EDIBLE, DELICIOUS

Craterellus cornucopioides
("small cup"   "horn of plenty")

COMMON NAMES

Horn of plenty, trumpet of death, cornucopia fungus, death trumpet, fairy's loving cup, fairy trumpet.

WHAT IT LOOKS LIKE

Cap: 1 to 3 inches across; trumpet- or funnel-shaped, looks like empty cornucopia to some; hollow to the base; trumpet interior gray-brown. *Flesh:* very thin, dingy brown, about the same color as the cap's interior surface. *Spore-producing Surface:* smooth to slightly wrinkled to slight imprint of veins, ash gray to blackish, "frosted;" looks like inside of a bicycle tire tube. *Stem:* ¾ to 2 inches tall; no sheen or powder as in frosted part of cap. *Spores:* pale buff. Mushroom is 2 to 4, sometimes 5, inches high.

KEY FEATURES

The trumpet shape, gray to blackish color, smooth to slightly wrinkled undersurface, and growth in large clusters are very distinctive. Another *Craterellus* species, *Craterellus fallax*, resembles the horn of plenty, except that the spore color of this species is a deeper yellow-brown. Mycologists also note a few other differences at the microscopic level, which don't concern us here. Because both species are edible and equally delicious, don't worry about trying to distinguish between the two species based on spore color. The general distinctive features mentioned above are sufficient.

WHERE FOUND

Grows in small groups or in large numbers on the ground in hardwoods or mixed forests. Found in eastern North America and along the Pacific Coast. Forms tufts on the woodland floor. Though common, the horn of plenty is difficult to see at first.

WHEN

Appears in summer and into fall.

Sulphur Shelf Mushroom

(Polyporus sulphureus)

Among the shadows of late summer, large splashes of bright orange and yellow may suddenly greet a woodland traveler. These spots of color festoon logs, form clusters that march up the bole of trees, and skirt the base of stumps (Figure 10 and Color Plate 10A). At a distance a careless eye may mistake these colorful objects as fallen leaves that prematurely herald the arrival of fall by turning color earlier than usual. However, closeup each of these bright objects turns out to be an unusually large fungus, appropriately called the sulphur shelf mushroom (*Polyporus sulphureus*), for the bright yellow underside of the caps (Color Plate 10B).

The sulphur shelf is one of the "foolproof four" designated by C. M. Christensen in his book *Common Edible Mushrooms*. "The shape and color make it impossible to confuse this species with any other mushroom," says Dr. Christensen. The beautiful sulphur shelf has a series of fan-shaped caps that look like overlapping petals of a large multicolored rose. On the top of each "petal" are bands of orange and yellow (Figure 11).

On the underside of the mushroom, the pores are a bright yellow that rivals the brilliant color of hot sulphur brine. In nine-teenth-century France, the distinctive color of this woodland fungus

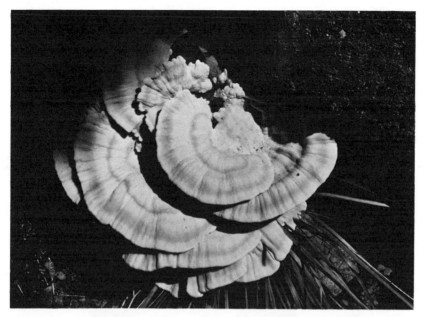

FIGURE 10. *Sulphur shelf* (Polyporus sulphureus) *at the base of a tree.*

was so appealing to the French clothiers, that they obtained a yellow dye from the mushroom for their material.

To scientists with a penchant for classification, the sulphur shelf is a *polypore*. Polypores are a group of fungi that have many tiny openings or pores on the underside of the mushroom. Polypores grow on wood and are usually tough to woody. The artist's fungus on which generations of people have carved initials or scratched drawings is an example of a woody polypore. Not all polypores are tough. Some, such as the sulphur shelf, are very tender and delicious.

The polypores are similar to boletes (see p. 136). Although the boletes also have a porous underside, they resemble the typical mushroom in that they have a cap and central stem. The fleshy boletes almost always grow on the ground, whereas the polypores are found on wood.

A sulphur shelf can grow to a large size: a clump the size of a basketball is not uncommon. Stacks of sulphur shelf may also form a line 20 feet up a tree. "I have seen at least a hundred pounds of it at one time on an old oak log, all fresh and inviting, and ready for the oven," William Alphonso Murrill, an early

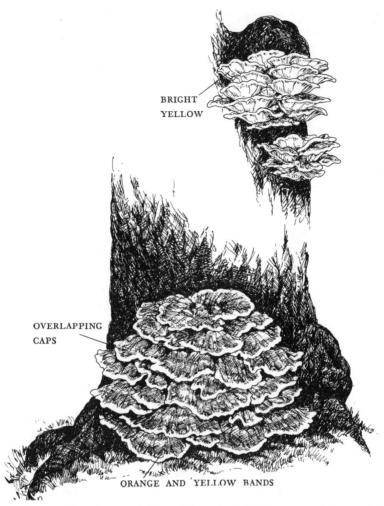

BRIGHT
YELLOW

OVERLAPPING
CAPS

ORANGE AND YELLOW BANDS

FIGURE 11. *Key features of a sulphur shelf* (Polyporus sulphureus).

twentieth-century American mycologist gleefully wrote. In an article in the July, 1929, issue of *Scientific American*, Murrill stumped for a more widespread appreciation of the culinary merits of this colorful stump mushroom. The article was appropriately entitled "Neglected Mushrooms." Fifty years later, I (and others) extoll this edible fungus.

The sulphur shelf is world-wide in distribution, being found in such diverse places as the Black Forest in Germany, the woodlands of the Far East, the deciduous forests of eastern United

States, and among the stately evergreens of the Pacific Northwest. The fungus has been recorded growing on more than one hundred different kinds of trees. Most of these species are hardwoods, such as oak, hickory, and ash. The mushroom generally begins fruiting in midsummer and may be found into fall. On several occasions, I have found the sulphur shelf fruiting in the spring.

The growth habit of the sulphur shelf may not always accommodate the edible mushroom seeker. It is frustrating to discover one or several sulphur shelves on a tree just above your reach. Armed with only a basket, you may stare longingly at the sulphur-colored caps on a branchless tree bole. A few swipes with a long stick may produce mixed results. However, other people have come up with more imaginative solutions.

A neighbor of mine was surprised to see a lineman from a local power company clamber rapidly up a dying tree. His crampon spikes sent slivers of wood flying as they dug into the tree for support. High in the leafless tree, the lineman plucked the object of his efforts, climbed back down, and drove off with his prize. It was a large sulphur shelf.

The sulphur shelf mushroom occupies an important place in the ecology of a woodland. It helps recycle trees back to the soil by breaking down or decaying the wood. The sulphur shelf attacks the *heartwood* of a tree. The heartwood is the solid center of the tree that is no longer alive. The heartwood, which in cross section shows up as the darker center of the familiar tree rings, provides most of the structural support for the outside, or growing part, of the tree. To reach the heartwood, a sulphur shelf fungus must find a chink in the protective bark of the tree. A lesion caused by lightning, a winter storm that broke off a branch, and a woodpecker hammering away, all provide openings for fungus spores to enter a tree. Once inside, the spores form a mycelium that permeates the heartwood. Enzymes from the mycelia attack and digest the wood cellulose, causing the wood to rot. As it rots, the wood becomes brown and cracks into many small pieces. Periodically, a fruiting body may appear at the spot where the spores were admitted. Eventually the wood, saturated by the mycelia, may become so rotted that it changes to powder when the wood is rubbed between the fingers.

Weakened of its support, a tree will eventually fall.

When a sulphur shelf invades a tree not coveted by humans, its destructiveness may be viewed as a natural recycling process. However, when the fungus attacks woodland trees that are to be marketed for timber, the fungus becomes a "pest." According to one U.S. Forest Service study, the sulphur shelf causes nearly $50 million worth of damage each year to hickory forests in Ohio, Kentucky, Indiana, Illinois, and Missouri.

The destructiveness of the sulphur shelf has also provided a mycological footnote to the early history of our country. When the Pilgrims were ready to set sail for America in 1620, they were originally scheduled to come over in two merchant ships, the *Mayflower* and the *Speedwell*. However, the *Speedwell* had to remain behind because its hull had become too rotted to safely traverse the Atlantic. According to John Ramsbottom, an eminent British mycologist who has made a lifetime study of mushroom lore, the sulphur shelf and a few other fungi were responsible for the damage.

In the early days of sailing, wood rotting caused by a host of fungi was a major problem. Trees containing the mycelia of the sulphur shelf mushroom and other fungi were often cut and used as ship-building material before they were properly seasoned (dried). Once part of a ship, the wood was subjected to alternating periods of wetting and drying. Coupled with the poor ventilation in the holds, conditions were ideal for the growth of the destructive mycelia. The problem became so severe that new ships literally rotted at their moorings before reaching the open sea. When Samuel Pepys, in his capacity as member of the Admiralty Board, made an inspection of thirty new ships of the British Navy in 1684, he was appalled by what he saw. Planks were "in many places perish'd to powder," the rotted ship's sides were patched by new planks, and, says Pepys, "I have with my own hand gather'd Toadstools growing, in the most considerable of them, as big as my Fist."

Even today, weekend sailors have cause to worry about the effects of the sulphur shelf. According to Dr. Ramsbottom, the fungus that altered *Speedwell*'s course in history is still plaguing all manner of wooden boats from lifeboats to yachts, speedboats, and even larger vessels. So if you see a bright yellow-orange object protruding from your best friend's yacht, try to break the news gently.

The sulphur shelf mushroom is one of the best edible mushrooms. Early American Indians boiled the mushroom and considered it a choice food. More recently, an informal survey was conducted among members of the New York Mycological Society by club member Emil Brand. The members were asked to rank their favorite mushrooms on an ABCD scale, with A their favorite mushroom, B their next favorite, and so on. The sulphur shelf came out on top.

Despite its rating on the edibility scale, some persons in California have reported mild digestive upsets when eating this mushroom raw or cooked (see p. 33). The indigestion may have been due to eating tougher parts of the mushroom or by eating a mildly toxic form, which may be present in that region, even though countless other people have eaten this mushroom in California and other parts of the country without ill effect. To rule out any possible problem, sauté and sample a small tender piece of the mushroom. If you do not experience any adverse reaction, you can eat the mushroom in larger amounts. Always eat only the most tender part of the mushroom.

When the sulphur shelf mushroom is very young, the entire fungus can be eaten. As it gets older, it becomes harder. Only the tender outer growing edges of the mushroom "petals" are then best to eat. A simple knife test will quickly determine the sulphur shelf's edibility. When the knife passes through the mushroom as effortlessly as if you were cutting through butter, the mushroom is tender enough to eat. If you meet resistance to the cutting, then that mushroom or part of the mushroom has passed its prime. I have often found a sulphur shelf so young that the entire mushroom felt like a slab of butter when I cut through it. Yet the mushroom at that time was about the size of a small basketball.

Many mushroom collectors return to the same mushroom again and again for more cuttings. By removing only the outer inch or so of the fungus "petals," the mushroom will continue to send out new tender growth that can be eaten.

The sulphur shelf, also commonly known as the chicken of the woods because of its resemblance to a sitting hen, is definitely the mushroom counterpart of the barnyard fowl. The mushroom tastes like chicken and the interior even looks like white chicken meat when it is broken up into small strips. Margaret Morris, a Long Island, New York, mushroom buff, recalls the time she served a casserole of sulphur shelf mushrooms at a garden club meeting. One member later congratulated the chef. However, the woman was apparently still squeamish about eating wild mushrooms, and confessed that she had "eaten all the chicken but left the rest." The chicken that she ate, of course, was the sulphur shelf.

Some people freeze large pieces of sulphur shelf mushrooms after blanching them in salted water. It's one of the few mushrooms that can be frozen this way and still taste good when removed from the freezer a few months later. One tree may supply enough sulphur shelf for an entire winter's supply in a freezer. Other people prefer to sauté the sulphur shelf pieces before freezing. Some people even freeze the mushroom without blanching or sautéing.

Sulphur shelf is good in casseroles, with eggs, or in almost any recipe as a substitute for chicken.

10 Sulphur Shelf Mushroom   Edible, Delicious

Polyporus sulphureus
("many pores"   "sulphur")

COMMON NAMES

Chicken fungus, chicken mushroom, chicken of the woods, sulphur polypore, sulphur shelf mushroom, sulphurous mushroom.

WHAT IT LOOKS LIKE

Fruiting Body: large clump or rosette up to 2 feet across at base of tree or stumps; caps can form overlapping shelves up side of tree or along log or stump; fanlike caps, 2 to 10 inches wide, bright orange to yellow bands on top, fade with age to paler color, sulphur-yellow pores below (see Color Plate 10B), pores are very small.

Flesh: white, pliable; looks like white chicken meat; tender at edge, tougher toward center in older specimens. *Spores:* white.

KEY FEATURES

There is no other species that has a bright sulphur-colored underside with clusters of overlapping orange-yellow caps. A less abundant variety of the sulphur shelf (*subalbinus*) has a white instead of a bright sulphur-colored undersurface.

WHERE FOUND

Grows on stumps, rotting logs, and from wounds of a living tree throughout the United States. Many may grow on one log.

WHEN

Typically late summer and fall, sometimes earlier.

Teeth Fungus

(*Hericium* and *Dentinum*)

SATYR'S BEARD (*Hericium erinaceus*)
BEAR'S HEAD FUNGUS (*Hericium ramosum*)
CORAL HYDNUM (*Hericium coralloides*)
HEDGEHOG MUSHROOM (*Dentinum repandum*)
SLENDER-STEMMED HEDGEHOG MUSHROOM
  (*Dentinum umbilicatum*)

The teeth fungi are an unusual group of mushrooms. The aptly named fungi can be easily identified by the teethlike spines or "icicles" that hang in large masses from the mushrooms (Figure 12). The spores are formed on these spines, representing one of the more unusual ways in which spores are disseminated in the world of fungi. The huge number of spines on these mushrooms has triggered a number of common names for this group of mushrooms, including hedgehog mushroom, spine fungi, coral fungus, and satyr's beard.

The teeth fungi are a diverse group. Many have a cap and stem and grow on the ground. When viewed from above, these mushrooms resemble a gilled mushroom. However, as soon as you peek under the cap, downward-pointing spines or teeth can be seen. Two ground-inhabiting tooth fungi, the spreading hydnum or hedgehog mushroom (*Dentinum repandum*) and the slender-stemmed hedgehog mushroom (*Dentinum umbilicatum*) are described in this section. Many people rank hedgehog mushrooms

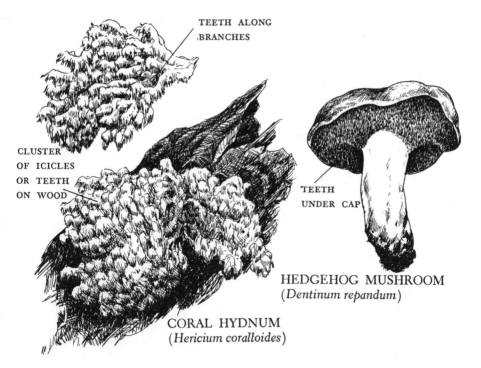

TEETH ALONG
BRANCHES

CLUSTER
OF ICICLES
OR TEETH
ON WOOD

TEETH
UNDER CAP

HEDGEHOG MUSHROOM
(*Dentinum repandum*)

CORAL HYDNUM
(*Hericium coralloides*)

FIGURE 12. *Key features of two kinds of teeth fungi, the* Hericium *and* Dentinum. *The coral hydnum has teeth that hang along the entire branches. The hedgehog mushroom has the cap and stem of a gilled mushroom and a white-spore deposit like that of the* Hericium.

among the top edibles along with the king bolete, morel, and chanterelle.

Some teeth fungi also form beautiful large clusters of white spines about the size of a small cauliflower on logs, stumps, and living trees. These species are very distinctive. All of these white mushrooms (*Hericium*) are edible, easy to identify, and are ideal mushrooms for beginners. One, the satyr's beard, truly looks like a white beard. Another, the bear's head fungus, forms an irregularly shaped cluster of tufts of white iciclelike spines. A third, the aptly named coral hydnum, branches like a coral with curtains of spines hanging from the branches. To come across one of these fungi festooning a log in the woodlands is a most beautiful experience.

The satyr's beard (*Hericium erinaceus*) is named for the bearded, part-human, part-animal Greek god Pan who roamed the

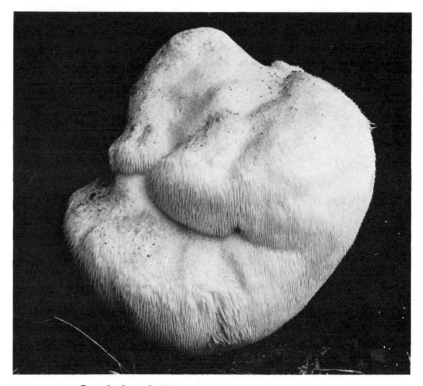

FIGURE 13. *Satyr's beard* (Hericium erinaceus).

woods. Spines 1 to 3 inches long crowd together in a dense, beard-like mass (Figure 13). The spines hang in parallel lines from a mass of tissue attached to a tree. The fungus has no branches. *Hericium erinaceus* ranges in size from 2 to 8 inches in diameter and grows from the wounds of living hardwood trees such as oak and beech. It may also be found on dead trees. A dead beech was once discovered covered on one side from root to crown with clumps of satyr's beard. The long spines of these fungi waved with each passing wind. At least 50 pounds of mushroom were collected from the tree. The satyr's beard is found in late summer and fall in the eastern and central United States and in Pacific Coast states.

The bear's head fungus is supposedly named for the small heads or tufts of spines that decorate this fungus (Figure 14). I fail to see the comparison. To me, the tufts look more like a series of small bearded cascades. These long flowing spines grow at the tips

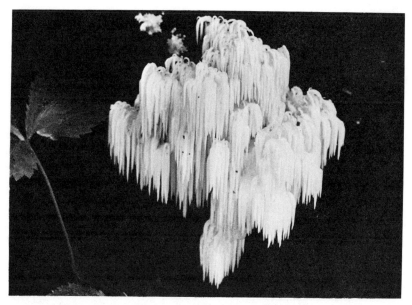

FIGURE 14. *Bear's head fungus* (Hericium ramosum).

of short branches mostly hidden by the dense curtain of spines. The bear's head fungus (*Hericium ramosum*) forms compact white clumps up to a foot in diameter on either evergreen or deciduous trees. Several of the large fruiting bodies may be found on one log or stump. Like the other *Hericium* species, the widely distributed bear's head fruits in late summer and fall.

The third white hericium is the coral hydnum, perhaps the most beautiful of the three white-spined species (Figure 12 and Color Plate 11). Arising from a short, white "trunk" attached to a tree or log, this fungus repeatedly branches into long slender shoots that form corallike clusters. The spines hang like icicles from the entire underside of the branches, not just at the branch tips as in the bear's head fungus. The appearance of this gorgeous, snow-white mushroom (*Hericium coralloides*) on a log in the woods never ceases to impress. In 1806, Elias Fries, a reknowned Swedish botanist who helped lay the groundwork for mycology by setting up a classification system for fungi, decided to devote his life to the study of fungi after spotting a coral hydnum while blueberry-ing with his mother as a child. Even when he wrote his auto-biography *Historiola Studii Mei Mycologici* fifty years later, Fries still vividly remembered the emotion that seized him when he found an unusually large specimen of the coral hydnum. That enthusiasm has been shared by the American mycologist Louis C. Kreiger. "This startlingly beautiful *Hydnum*," he wrote in *The Mushroom Handbook*, "its pure whiteness seen in contrast with the dark colors of some fallen, moss-covered monarch of the forest, will cause even the most callous to stop in wonder and admiration. It seems almost sacrilegious to recommend it as food for the camper who wishes to vary his diet with a taste of mushrooms. Let him turn to the more humble kinds to satisfy his craving for something to eat, and reserve this glorious *Hydnum* for a feast of the eye." Although you can agree with Kreiger about the beauty of the coral hydnum, don't be deterred from tasting the mushroom as well. It's one of the safest mushrooms for a beginner.

A white *Hericium* is considered a prize find by collectors. Because of its large size, one of these mushrooms can provide enough for at least one meal. Collect *Hericium* species only when they are young, white, and firm. Do not gather species whose tips have begun to turn yellow or brown. These fungi are too old and tough; the yellow or brown colors indicate that the *Hericium* is drying out and beginning to disintegrate.

The one exception to this change-in-color rule is *Hericium abietis*, a generally rare species that grows on conifers in the Pacific Northwest in the fall. Unlike the other three *Hericia*, *Hericium abietis* has a yellowish color when young instead of white. Its color varies from yellowish orange to buff in youth, becoming paler in age. This large mushroom, which can grow up to 30 inches high, forms a thick mass from which short branches covered with short teeth emerge. *Hericium abietis* is edible and good and is commonly collected. However, beginners in the Pacific Northwest, on the remote chance that they would confuse this yellowish mushroom with an old white *Hericium* species that has turned yellow, should probably collect only *Hericia* that are white.

The three white-toothed fungi are generally considered good to very good in taste. The mild-tasting mushrooms can be sautéed in butter and served with vegetables. *Hericium* may also be used in Chinese recipes as a substitute for bean sprouts, which have a similar texture.

Occasionally *Hericium* may have a slightly bitter taste. If this is the case, parboil the mushroom, drain, and sauté in butter before serving as a vegetable or using in a recipe.

Another spined mushroom that is a favorite of many is the hedgehog mushroom (*Dentinum repandum*). While collectors looking for a white *Hericium* always focus their search on some standing or fallen wood, the hedgehog mushroom is found on the ground in woodlands. The hedgehog mushroom has a cap and stem like a gilled mushroom (Color Plate 12), but its underside is filled with hundreds of spines that look like canine teeth, the spines of a hedgehog, or the bristles of a rubber brush. The uneven, velvety cap is large, from 3 to 6 inches in diameter, and varies in color from orange to cream to tan or even reddish tan-brown. The chunky stipe is white or colored like the cap, and the teeth are whitish to cream-colored.

The hedgehog mushroom begins to appear toward the end of summer and becomes more frequent as fall approaches. It continues fruiting into October. If the summer season is unusually wet, the mushroom may appear as early as July. The mushroom matures slowly and remains fresh and edible longer than most mushrooms. (The thick, white flesh is rather brittle.)

The hedgehog mushroom grows commonly throughout the United States. It is found singly or sometimes in small clusters under hardwoods or evergreens. The fungus grows in leaf duff, on bare soil, and around wood that has been greatly decayed. Although the mushroom is common, you rarely find large numbers growing close together in a small area. The mushroom tends to grow more scattered throughout the woodland. When I'm making a mushroom meal, I sometimes combine the mushroom with others that I have collected during a late summer foray.

A diminutive version of the hedgehog mushroom, also edible, is usually found along the edges of swamps and bogs in eastern North America. The slender-stemmed hedgehog mushroom (*Dentinum umbilicatum*), as the name suggests, has a thinner stalk

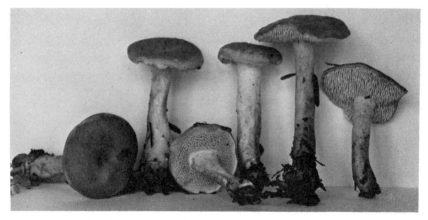

FIGURE 15. *Slender-stemmed hedgehog mushroom* (Dentinum umbilicatum).

(about pencil-size) than the hedgehog mushroom, is smaller, and is usually dimpled in the center of the cap (Figure 15). The Latin name for the mushroom means umbilicus (navel), which refers to the cap's depression. The cap is orange-brown to reddish brown and is sometimes darker in the center than around the edge. The stem is paler than the cap, becoming darkened when bruised. The spores are white. The mushroom grows under evergreens, especially cedar, balsam, and spruce.

Although the stem of the hedgehog mushroom (*Dentinum repandum*) varies in width (see Color Plate 12 and Figure 12), it never narrows to the width of a pencil as it does in the slender-stemmed hedgehog mushroom (Figure 15). Both species are delicious and are often collected together. While the hedgehog mushroom begins appearing in summer, the slender-stemmed species is most abundant after heavy rains in September.

There are other teeth fungi that grow on the ground. However, most are too tough to eat or have an extremely bitter taste. The distinctive orange to cream-colored hedgehog mushroom has a mild taste when fresh and is not tough. Among the teeth fungi, limit your collecting to the hedgehog mushroom and *Dentinum umbilicatum* among the ground dwellers and to the three white *Hericia* among the wood dwellers.

Dentinum repandum compares favorably with any mushroom in taste and can be used in almost any mushroom dish. Because the thick firm mushroom has a texture similar to that of the chanterelle, it can be used in chanterelle recipes as well. The mushroom also goes well with lamb or oysters. The hedgehog mushroom can be preserved by drying. Before drying, the mushroom should be sliced into thin pieces. The dried slices smell inviting even one to two years later. These comments apply to the slender-stemmed hedgehog mushroom as well.

11 Coral Hydnum EDIBLE, GOOD

Hericium coralloides
("hedgehog" "corallike")

COMMON NAMES
Coral hydnum, coral fungus.

WHAT IT LOOKS LIKE
Fruiting body: large, variable in size; usually 4 to 8 inches across, sometimes even much larger, white; a mass of corallike branches arises from a short white trunk; smaller branches covered with iciclelike or stalactitelike white teeth, about 1 inch long; teeth grow from underside of branches; branches taper to point, with a filigree of spines. *Flesh:* white. *Spores:* white.

KEY FEATURES
A white, corallike growth on logs with spines hanging from underside of branches.

WHERE FOUND
Widely distributed on logs or stumps in the western coastal states, central United States, and the Northeast. Fir, oak, and beech are some of the trees on which this beautiful fungus grows. A large log of beech is a favorite habitat. A moist season may yield several crops from same tree.

WHEN

Late summer and fall.

12 Hedgehog Mushroom   EDIBLE, DELICIOUS
Dentinum repandum
("teeth"   "bent backward")

COMMON NAMES

Hedgehog mushroom, spreading hydnum.

WHAT IT LOOKS LIKE

Cap: 2 to 6 inches across; convex becoming nearly flat in age; cream to orange to tan with a hint of red; feels like kid glove; edge of cap wavy, somewhat bent back or turned upward in places. *Flesh:* thick, soft, brittle, white. *Teeth:* various lengths; tender; white to cream-colored. *Stem:* 2 to 5 inches tall; thick; colored like the cap or paler; solid; may be enlarged at base; sometimes covered with a white coating. *Spores:* white.

KEY FEATURES

A large cream- to orange-colored velvety mushroom with cream-colored teeth and a thick white to cream stipe distinguishes this fungus. A nearly white variety occurs in the fall, whereas the more colorful variety begins appearing in the summer. The whiter variety is identical except in color.

WHERE FOUND

Grows in hardwoods and evergreen forests as well as in mixtures of both. Grows throughout the United States and Canada. In the western states, the large, nearly white variety is most widely collected.

WHEN

Late summer and fall.

Meadow Mushroom

(*Agaricus campestris*)

Rodman's Mushroom

(*Agaricus bitorquis*)

Toward the end of summer when rains become more frequent, a short, stocky, white mushroom with pink to chocolate-brown gills appears on lawns, pastures, fields, and golf courses. This is (*Agaricus campestris*), the meadow mushroom (Figure 16), a close relative of the common cultivated white mushroom found in supermarkets. The Latin name for the meadow mushroom, *campestris*, clearly shows the fungus's preference for open areas; the word means "pertaining to fields." The meadow mushroom will never be found in the woods. Instead, it grows in scattered groups of several mushrooms or forms partial circles or fairy rings. The rings or arcs may be quite large as the mushroom mycelia grow outward each year from a central spot, and the fruiting bodies spring upward from the leading edge of the ever-widening circle. The mushrooms often seem to be all cap and no bottom because the stipe is so short. The cap does not rise much higher than blades of grass on a lawn, and in a meadow, the grass may actually be taller than the mushroom.

The meadow mushroom goes through various stages of growth. The cycle begins with the button stage, as a small round white button pushes its way up through the ground from the my-

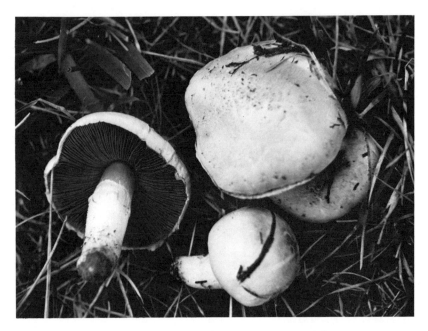

FIGURE 16. *Meadow mushroom* (Agaricus campestris).

celia. This button is the unopened cap of the meadow mushroom.
At this stage, the gills on the underside are covered by a cottony
veil. As the cap expands, the veil separates, revealing beautiful
pink gills. The chalk-white cap and stipe with drops of rain or
dew provide a delicate frame for the subtle pink gills. The con-
spicuous pink of the gills has resulted in another common name
for *Agaricus campestris*—the pink bottom (see Color Plate 13).

After the veil has separated from the cap, it forms a collar
on the stipe. This fragile collar is sometimes washed off by rain.
Bits of the veil may also cling to the edge of the cap, like a short
tattered curtain. Meanwhile, the gills of the cap turn from pink
to chocolate brown as they fill with dark brown spores. When
fully grown, the meadow mushroom may be 1 to 2½ inches high
with a cap up to 4 inches in diameter.

Despite the distinctive characteristics of the meadow mushroom, the careless viewer may confuse this mushroom with the
deadly white amanitas. Yet, other than sharing a cap that is white
and a collar or ring, the two types of mushrooms are really quite
distinctive (Figure 17). The gills of the meadow mushroom are

pink to chocolate brown; the gills of the amanitas are white. The meadow mushroom is *short* and *stocky;* the amanitas are *tall* and *stately.* The meadow mushroom has *no cuplike volva* at the base of the stipe; amanitas do *have a volva.* And finally, the meadow mushroom is an inhabitant of *open, grassy areas;* amanitas are most often found in *woods.* Although the last observation is generally true, care must be exercised because a stray white amanita may appear on the lawn at the edge of a woodland, or in grassy areas where trees are plentiful, or when a lawn has recently been created from a woodland area. The following guidelines should ensure that you never make a mistake while collecting meadow mushrooms.

(1) Dig out the base of the stipe with a knife to make sure no volva is present. Merely cutting the mushroom cap and part of the stipe is insufficient, because most of the volva is buried in the soil or humus. Be especially carefuly in checking the button stage for a volva.

(2) Collect only in grassy areas, such as fields, meadows, lawns, and golf courses.

(3) Make sure that the mushroom has pink to chocolate-brown gills and is short and chunky.

In addition to studying the key differences between the meadow mushroom and a white amanita (*Amanita virosa*) (see Figure 17 and Color Plates 13 and 14), you can also become familiar with the general characteristics of a meadow mushroom by studying its close relative, the cultivated white mushroom. Buy a box of the commercial white variety that contains the greatest number of mushroom growth stages. Note the pink to chocolate-brown gills, the chunky cap and stipe (which is partially cut off). Although the cultivated variety does differ slightly from the wild meadow mushroom, the resemblance is close enough so that you will have a clear idea of what you are looking for when you venture forth on your first trip.

Fortunately, the white amanitas do not grow in all regions of the United States. The six deadly white amanitas, known collectively as the destroying angels, grow in woodlands in eastern North America and on the other side of the continent in the Pacific Northwest and Pacific Coast states. To the naked eye all

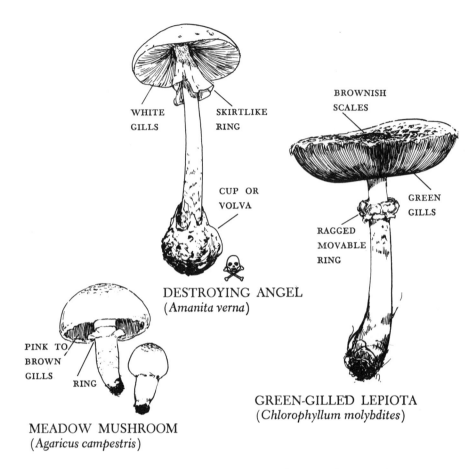

WHITE
GILLS

SKIRTLIKE
RING

BROWNISH
SCALES

CUP OR
VOLVA

GREEN
GILLS

RAGGED
MOVABLE
RING

DESTROYING ANGEL
(*Amanita verna*)

PINK TO
BROWN
GILLS

RING

GREEN-GILLED LEPIOTA
(*Chlorophyllum molybdites*)

MEADOW MUSHROOM
(*Agaricus campestris*)

FIGURE 17. *Key features of the stocky meadow mushroom* (Agaricus campestris) *and look-alikes, the all-white, tall destroying angel and the green-gilled lepiota. The skull and crossbones indicate that the species is deadly.*

have similar characteristics: tall white mushroom with white gills, a skirtlike ring, and a volva. Three of these white amanita species (*Amanita verna*, *Amanita virosa*, and *Amanita bisporigera*) fruit more commonly in eastern woodlands in the spring, summer, or fall. However, in the Pacific Northwest and coastal states, these species are rare, indicating that these mushrooms may not be native to the West. Perhaps they were introduced accidentally when trees with which they form mycorrhizae were transported westward. The three remaining species comprising the destroying angels are more limited in known distribution, being confined to only one state apiece. *Amanita tenuifolia* and *Amanita suballiacea* grow in Florida, while the sixth destroying angel, *Amanita ocreata*, is found in California under oaks.

A seventh deadly amanita, *Amanita phalloides*, differs from the white amanitas by having an olive-green cap. It is found in the Northeast and Mid-Atlantic states as far south as Virginia, and in the western coastal states.

Two other species of mushrooms that grow on lawns have sometimes been confused with the meadow mushroom. One of these species, which commonly appears in the southern states, is the green-gilled lepiota known to scientists as *Chlorophyllum molybdites* (Figure 17). Like the meadow mushroom, this mostly white species may form large fairy rings on pastures. However, this mushroom can be distinguished from the meadow mushroom by the greenish gills, the brownish scales that form on top of the large cap, and the tall stipe. It also has a ring with ragged edges, which can be moved up and down the stipe like a free collar. This fungus can grow to a large size with the cap sometimes reaching a foot in diameter. This mycological heavyweight shouldn't be confused with the chunkier meadow mushroom, but it sometimes is.

Another grassy inhabitant sometimes mistakenly identified as the meadow mushroom because of its white color and ring on the stem is the white lepiota (*Leucoagaricus naucina*). As with the amanitas, the white gills as well as its tallness quickly separate the white lepiota from the meadow mushroom. The white lepiota actually looks more like a white amanita than a meadow mushroom. However, it does not have a cuplike volva, and its ring is more like a round collar than a skirt. Its cap is egg-shaped. By simply avoiding tall, white mushrooms with white gills, you won't confuse this mushroom (or the amanitas) with the meadow mushroom.

Although many people eat both *Leucoagaricus naucina* and *Chlorophyllum molybdites*, having collected them for years without apparent effects, the mushrooms are known to be poisonous to some people. The white lepiota has caused mild to severe diarrhea in some individuals, while the green-gilled lepiota may cause nausea, vomiting, cramps, and diarrhea. In 1974, researchers F. I. Eilers and B. L. Barnard found that a toxin in *Chlorophyllum molybdites* became inactivated when heated in water at very high temperatures for a half hour. Thus persons who were poisoned by eating this mushroom may not have cooked it long enough. The best solution in such cases is to simply avoid eating the mushroom. By limiting yourself to short, chunky, white mushrooms that grow in grassy areas and have pink to chocolate-brown gills, you should be safe.

The only known exception to this general rule is a species of *Agaricus* mushroom that is found in a very limited area along the central and southern California coast. This species, appropriately named *Agaricus californicus*, grows on lawns and under trees in that region. Although considered edible for many years, this California mushroom has recently caused stomach upsets in some people. Although the mushroom does resemble a meadow mushroom in some ways, certain important characteristics set the two species apart. One of the most striking characteristics is that *Agaricus californicus* smells like Lysol or creosote. This odor is due to the presence of phenol (carbolic acid) in the mushroom. When the mushroom is cooked, the odor becomes even stronger.

Another important difference is the strong color change that occurs in *Agaricus californicus* when drops of water containing Drano (caustic soda) are added to the mushroom's surface. This Drano test causes the mushroom to turn a rich yellow where the drops were added. When the solution is added to the meadow mushroom, however, no color change is noted. Although other characteristics such as a rubbery ring (annulus) and a usually smoky brown cap may be used to help distinguish *Agaricus californicus* from *Agaricus campestris*, the Drano test is the best method (and is foolproof) for differentiating these two species that grow in grassy areas in California. Beginners who live in the California coastal region who wish to collect the meadow mushroom should carry in their basket a screw-top container containing a solution of Drano (proportion: 1 teaspoon Drano to ¼ cup water).

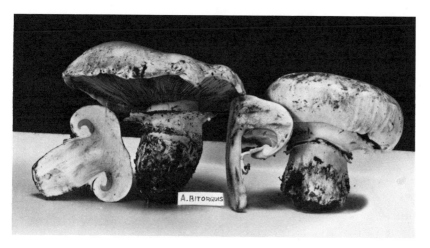

FIGURE 18. *Rodman's mushroom* (Agaricus bitorquis). *Note how the ring forms after the cap expands.*

The few seconds that it takes to prepare such a solution is worth the effort.

Throughout the United States, the meadow mushroom thrives especially well on fertilized lawns and in undisturbed pastures where cattle provide a rich source of nutrients. The appearance of the meadow mushroom is closely linked with the weather patterns of summer and fall. To fruit, the meadow mushroom seems to need a combination of cool nights and some rain. Such conditions usually begin in August, triggering the first prolific fruiting of the meadow mushroom. If the weather has been unusually cool and wet earlier in the summer, the mushrooms will fruit earlier. I have seen a few specimens as early as June, but these can be considered an aberration or tentative foray rather than the typical fruiting. Once the meadow mushroom makes its usual appearance in late summer, it will continue to fruit into fall, provided, of course, that there is enough precipitation. In some years, meadow mushrooms are much more abundant than in others. If the weather is too dry in summer and early fall, a sparse collection will result. A wet, cool period following a fairly dry summer seems to be ideal for fruiting. In seasons of abundant fruiting, meadow mushrooms will dot fields and lawns in such profusion that literally bushel baskets of these mushrooms can be collected. In some of these fields, only a few mushrooms may have been seen the previous year.

Another chunky, brown-spored mushroom, closely related to the meadow mushroom, is Rodman's mushroom (*Agaricus bitorquis*) (see Figure 18). Though not as common as *Agaricus campestris*, Rodman's mushroom seems to flourish on hard ground. It has been found on hard-packed soil around barnyards, old driveways, school yards, pathways in parks, in areas used by carnivals and circuses, in tennis courts, and in open patches of grassless areas in the middle of a city. This mushroom has also been seen forcing its way up through cement pavement. Its preference for hard-packed soil is borne out near the building where I work. Each year, I find meadow mushrooms growing in semicircles or in rings in different areas of the lawn. However, in one small, well-trafficked, bare spot, I can always find one or two Rodman's mushrooms. And the mushroom is only found there. The mushroom always fruits in this spot before the meadow mushrooms show up, appearing in June. Rodman's mushroom, though widely distributed, is most common in eastern North America. It appears most abundantly in the spring, in late summer and fall.

In addition to its favored habitat of hard-packed soil, the *Agaricus bitorquis* can be distinguished from *Agaricus campestris* by its chunkier stature, larger size, and double ring growing on the stipe. The term *double ring* means that the ring curls outward at the lower edge of the ring and flares outward at the upper edge. The ring is located about halfway up the stipe. The mushroom is exceptionally delicious. Its solid flesh keeps well and some mycologists think this species would make a better commercial mushroom than the *Agaricus bisporus* now used. There is great interest in Europe and in the United States in growing this mushroom commercially and, in fact, it has been grown from spawn by some growers.

The meadow mushroom is also a delicious mushroom. It is one of the few wild mushrooms that can be eaten raw in salads without concern. It has a stronger flavor than the commercial

Agaricus and can be used in any recipe calling for the cultivated mushroom.

The meadow mushroom is delicious in a steak sauce, in mushroom soup, and any other way you prepare the store-bought, cultivated mushroom. Interestingly, in the United States, Americans prefer the cultivated *Agaricus* when they are pink and at the button stage. Europeans favor more mature mushrooms with brown gills because the mushrooms are said to have more taste. In the wild, both the pink-gilled and the brown-gilled mushrooms are excellent.

To preserve the meadow mushroom, sauté, then freeze.

13 Meadow Mushroom   EDIBLE, DELICIOUS
Agaricus campestris
("of the country"   "fields")

COMMON NAMES

Meadow mushroom, pink bottom, field mushroom, cream puffs, pink undies, common mushroom, pasture mushroom.

WHAT IT LOOKS LIKE

Cap: generally 1 to 3 inches across, sometimes 4; convex, nearly flat when older; dry, smooth, sometimes hairy in age with white to brown threads; satiny white surface may become light brown when old. *Flesh:* thick, firm, white; unchanging in color when cut. *Gills:* delicate pink, changing to chocolate brown; gills are not connected to the stipe. *Stem:* short, 1 to 2½ inches tall, the same width along entire stem or tapers toward base; white, cottony ring, sometimes wearing off; stipe white and silky smooth above ring, white and fuzzy or hairier below; flesh, white, spongy or fibrous. *Spores:* chocolate brown.

KEY FEATURES

This short, stocky, white mushroom, with pink to chocolate-brown gills and a ring on its stipe, grows in grassy areas. To avoid confusing the species with the deadly amanitas or with the green-gilled lepiota or the white lepiota, simply remember the key features of the meadow mushroom, and avoid tall, white mushrooms with white or green gills and with a volva. For California coastal residents, an additional test with a Drano solution is needed to distinguish the meadow mushroom for *Agaricus californicus*. Rodman's mushroom, another Agaricus, is similar to the meadow mushroom, but is chunkier, grows in hard-packed soil and has a double ring. Because Rodman's mushroom is a choice edible, there is no problem if you mistake the meadow mushroom for this species.

WHERE FOUND
On lawns, golf courses, fields, meadows, and pastures throughout North America.

WHEN
Late summer and fall, although it may appear earlier in summer when weather is unusually cool and wet.

14 Destroying Angel   POISONOUS, DEADLY
Amanita virosa
("mushroom" "poisonous")

COMMON NAMES
Destroying angel, death angel, white amanita, poisonous amanita.

WHAT IT LOOKS LIKE
Cap: 2 to 5 inches across; at first cone- to egg-shaped, becoming convex to flat; smooth, sticky, pure white. *Flesh:* white. *Gills:* white, crowded, not attached to stem. *Stem:* 3 to 8 inches tall; white; saclike volva at base; skirtlike white ring; stem surface sometimes scaly. *Spores:* white.

KEY FEATURES

Tall, stately white mushroom with white gills, a skirtlike ring, and a volva at the base. Other deadly white amanitas have similar characteristics in the field and all are to be avoided.

WHERE FOUND

Grows under hardwoods or in mixed conifer and deciduous woodlands in eastern North America and the Pacific Coast.

WHEN

Summer and fall.

Puffball

(*Calvatia, Calbovista,* and *Lycoperdon*)

GIANT PUFFBALL (*Calvatia gigantea*)
WESTERN GIANT PUFFBALL (*Calvatia booniana*)
CUP-SHAPED PUFFBALL (*Calvatia cyathiformis*)
BRAIN PUFFBALL (*Calvatia craniformis*)
WARTED GIANT PUFFBALL (*Calbovista subsculpta*)
PEAR-SHAPED PUFFBALL (*Lycoperdon pyriforme*)
GEMMED PUFFBALL (*Lycoperdon perlatum*)

Puffballs are one of the safest and most easily recognized group of mushrooms for a beginner or expert collecting for the table. These mushrooms are usually round to pear-shaped, often very large, and do not have a stipe as many gilled mushrooms do. (Figure 19). The inside of the puffball, when mature, is filled with billions of spores that emerge when the outside wall of the mushroom splits or breaks open.

The general name for puffballs and their relatives, *Gastromycetes,* refers to the fact that the spore-bearing surface is inside the fruiting body. *Gastro* means "stomach," and *mykes* is the Greek word for "fungus." Because puffballs are so frequently seen on lawns, they are among the first mushrooms that people can identify. In late summer and early fall, puffballs about the size of softballs or round loaves of bread spring up on lawns, pastures, and along the edges of woodlands. Many a youth has given this mycological "football" a swift boot, only to be surprised as the mature mushroom issued a smoky cloud. The "smoke" was the

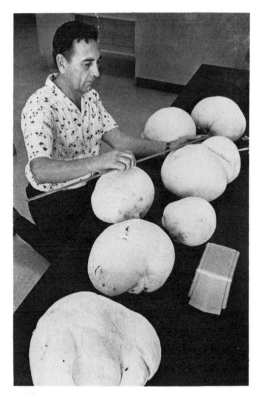

FIGURE 19. *Giant puffballs* (Calvatia gigantea), *being measured by Professor John Baxter of the University of Wisconsin, Milwaukee, show the typical round shape of these fungi.* Calvatia, *the Latin term for this group of puffballs, means bald.*

result of billions of spores leaving the puffball sooner than expected.

The spore output of puffballs is prodigious. A. H. R. Buller, a Canadian mycologist from the University of Manitoba, once calculated that a puffball 16 inches long, 12 inches wide, and 10 inches high would produce 7 trillion (7,000,000,000,000) spores. If each of these spores produced a puffball the same size as the parent, the combined mass of the puffballs would be 800 times the size of the earth. It must be pointed out, however, that very few of these spores mature into puffballs. Perhaps one out of every billion spores lands in a spot where conditions are right for spore development.

The goal of the puffball collector is to find a puffball before it reaches this advanced stage. You should look for a puffball that is entirely white inside when cut in half vertically and which has the consistency of cream cheese (Color Plate 17B). That's all you need to know to safely collect this common group of distinc-

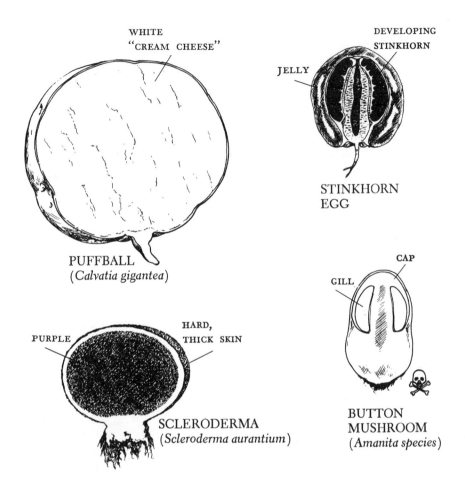

WHITE
"CREAM CHEESE"

DEVELOPING
STINKHORN

JELLY

STINKHORN
EGG

PUFFBALL
(*Calvatia gigantea*)

CAP

GILL

HARD,
THICK SKIN

PURPLE

SCLERODERMA
(*Scleroderma aurantium*)

BUTTON
MUSHROOM
(*Amanita species*)

FIGURE 20. *Cross sections of edible puffball and look-alikes.*

tively shaped mushrooms. At this young growth stage, the puffball
is edible and very good. Later, as the spores develop, the mushroom's interior becomes mustard-yellow, brown, or purple as it
turns powdery; it also becomes inedible. At the final stage of spore
development, your meal literally goes up in smoke.

If you slice a puffball in half from top to bottom and find an
entirely white, cream-cheese-like interior, you have ruled out any
possible mistake in identification. For example, stinkhorn eggs, a
young stage of a foul-smelling mushroom, may resemble puffballs
(see Figure 20). But as soon as one of these eggs is cut in half, the
difference is obvious. The interior of a stinkhorn egg is filled with

a clear jelly and the outline of a developing mushroom. A strong odor can also be noted.

Once you encounter these rubbery, smelly eggs, a warning not to eat them will seem superfluous. Although Charles Mc-Ilvaine, with his universal taste, claims that stinkhorn eggs are good when fried, there have been recent instances of curious children who have become poisoned after eating some species of stinkhorns.

In any case, it is wise to slice a puffball in half to make sure that you do not have the button stage of a poisonous mushroom. If a button gilled mushroom is cut from top to bottom, the cross section of an immature cap, stalk, and gills will be readily seen. If this undeveloped mushroom is white, then you may be observing the button stage of a deadly amanita. Do not collect any mushroom whose interior contains a developing cap or gills. Stay with a mushroom that has a uniform, white, cream-cheese-like interior.

This guideline also will help you to distinguish between the common edible puffballs and a thick-skinned, very hard group of puffballs known as earthballs or *Sclerodermas.* The Latin name for this group means "hard skin." Sclerodermas are extremely solid, almost rocklike, puffballs; in most species the interior quickly turns purple to black when cut (Figure 20 and Color Plate 18). A tough outer skin, like the rind of a dried orange, surrounds the solid interior. At the very youngest stage, a scleroderma interior may be a dull white. However, it is as hard as the inside of a potato, whereas the common edible puffballs are spongy. For every white scleroderma that I find, I usually will discover ten whose interior has already become purple or black. A simple press test will quickly separate the sclerodermas from the other puffballs. If you press down on the tough outer surface of a developing scleroderma with your thumb or finger, you will barely make a dent. If you do this with the soft, edible puffballs, you will easily poke a hole through the surface.

Avoid eating sclerodermas. They have a bitter taste, and some people have reported digestive upsets after eating them.

Edible puffballs may be conveniently divided into two main

groups: the large puffballs (*Calvatia* and *Calbovista*) and the smaller, often pear-shaped puffballs (mostly *Lycoperdons*). A gastronomic (not a scientific) separation between the two groups would be that a large puffball provides enough food for a meal—often for an entire family—whereas the smaller puffballs have to be collected like grapes to provide a meal.

The large puffballs often grow to a huge size and include several record holders among mushrooms. One of the largest puffballs is appropriately called the giant puffball (*Calvatia gigantea*). This popular edible mushroom (Color Plate 15) is usually found along the edges of meadows, near small streams or drainage ditches, or along old roads. The large size and smooth white surface of the puffball makes it stand out wherever it is found. Although specimens a foot or so in diameter and weighing several pounds are common, giant puffballs also grow much larger. Specimens 2 feet across and weighing more than 40 pounds have also been found. In 1877, a record-sized puffball was discovered in New York State. The puffball was 5 feet 4 inches long, 4 feet 6 inches wide, and 9½ inches high; its circumference was about 15½ feet! The puffball was so huge that from a distance it was mistaken for a sheep.

Such mushrooms, of course, do not spring up overnight. It takes about two weeks for a large puffball to reach maturity. Studies made by an early New York State botanist, C. H. Peck, showed that the girth of a large puffball swells at a rate of about 3 to 4 inches a day.

Another large common puffball is the cup-shaped puffball (*Calvatia cyathiformis*), a familiar inhabitant of lawns and pastures (Color Plate 17A and B). This puffball obtained its popular name because of the cuplike, papery base that remains after a spore eruption has blown most of the mushroom away.

The cup-shaped puffball, when still intact, is about the size of a large softball. It is much larger on top, tapering toward a thick base. To me, it often looks like a nearly round loaf of bread. In fact, if you cut off a slice of the puffball from top to bottom, the piece will look like a slice of bread. The surface of the cup-shaped puffball varies from whitish to pinkish tan and feels like kid gloves. Several of these puffballs grow in a circle or fairy ring on my lawn. I know exactly where to look for the mushrooms even before they come up. A rich circle of deep green grass marks the site of the ever-widening fairy ring. The cup-shaped puffballs emerge on the outer edge of the ring.

I begin looking for this puffball in August, after heavy rains. The puffball continues to be plentiful when the town fairs blossom throughout the New England countryside in September. I sometimes collect a few on the way home from a fair to simplify the evening's cooking after an active day.

The cup-shaped puffball (or any other mushroom) does not necessarily appear on the same day in every location in the area. Local conditions such as availability of nutrients and slight differences in miniclimate may alter the time schedule of a puffball's emergence. Cup-shaped puffballs often spring up on someone's lawn on the other side of town after the puffballs on my fairy ring have been collected and eaten. And so one must seek greener pastures (or lawns) to replenish one's supply. A friend of mine admits that he sneaks out early on weekend mornings to forage on his neighbors' lawns. I once had another solution.

My family and I used to cruise the town in the car, scanning the lawns for puffballs. When a crop was spotted, one of the three children (who had become quite adept at spotting mushrooms) would give a yell. I would stop the car, and while the engine ran (this was before the energy crisis), a child would hop out to scoop up the puffball or puffballs. As he scrambled back, a second child would close the door, and away we would go with the bounty.

Another puffball that resembles the cup-shaped puffball is the brain or skull-shaped puffball (*Calvatia craniformis*) (Figure 21). The large top is wrinkled like the folds of a brain, and the mushroom tapers downward toward the base. This large puffball is just as edible as the other large puffballs when the interior is white. Unlike the cup-shaped puffball, which grows in open, grassy areas, the brain puffball is usually found in the woods and in brushy areas. I have found it more common later in the puffball season, after the growth of *Calvatia cyathiformis*.

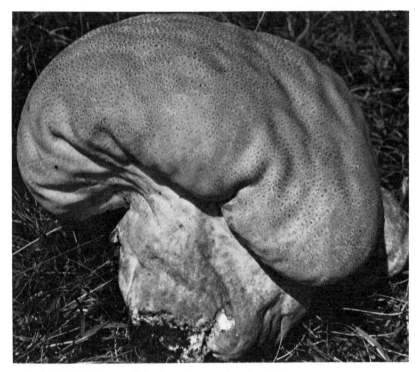

FIGURE 21. *Brain puffball* (Calvatia craniformis).

The brain puffball is about the same size as the cup-shaped puffball. When the puffball is mature, its interior changes to a greenish yellow or yellow-brown, whereas in *Calvatia cyathiformis* the interior becomes purple-brown.

Not all large puffballs ready to be collected have the smooth youthful chamoislike feel and appearance as the three *Calvatias* already mentioned. The Latin word itself means "bald" and refers to the smooth surface of many of these puffballs. In the West, there are large, edible puffballs that have a rougher or cracked surface even though the interior of the puffball is still a soft, uniform white throughout.

One such species is the western giant puffball (*Calvatia booniana*). This egg-shaped, dull white to tan puffball with a rough (later cracked) surface (Color Plate 16) grows in dry, open areas of the West. It may be found after heavy summer rains under sagebrush, near old corrals, and in other arid habitats. This

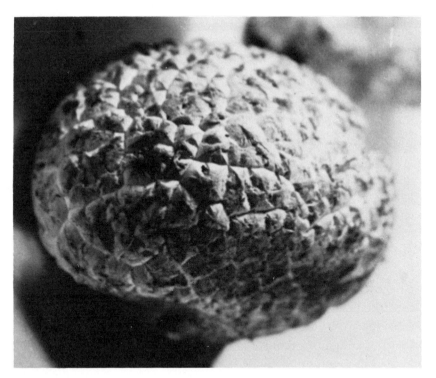

FIGURE 22. *Warted giant puffball* (Calbovista subsculpta)

is the giant puffball that many westerners have collected and eaten since pioneer days.

Another common, large, edible western mushroom (Figure 22) is the warted giant puffball (*Calbovista subsculpta*). Unlike the western giant puffball, this mushroom prefers the higher, cooler elevations of the West. It usually grows in or near evergreen mountain forests. The puffball is covered with low warts that look like pyramids with their tops shaven off. Brownish hairs are in the center of these cone-shaped warts. The mushroom near its base is often smooth to wrinkled but not warted.

The warted giant puffball is about the size of a softball, although in wet seasons it may be much larger. Shaped like a flattened egg, the white *Calbovista subsculpta* has an interior that changes from white to dark brown when the spores mature. In the high altitudes of the Rockies and coast ranges, the mushroom may appear as early as late spring. It is also found throughout the summer. It's a common western puffball.

Another puffball, *Calvatia sculpta,* is similar to the giant warted puffball except that its cones or pyramids are very long and pointed, and not truncated. This spectacular spiny puffball is found at higher elevations in the Rocky Mountains, Pacific Northwest, and Pacific Southwest. It is also very good.

The easy availability of the large puffballs in my area has spoiled me so that I do not bother collecting the smaller puffballs which other people enjoy eating. These puffballs (mostly *Lycoperdons,* which means "send forth into the air") are about the size and shape of golf balls or small pears. The small puffballs are widely distributed throughout the United States, growing in such diverse habitats as golf courses, lawns, rich woodland soil, and on logs. The small size of these mushrooms is dramatically illustrated by the fact that golfers continually mistake *Lycoperdons* on the fairways for golfballs. This lack of size is more than compensated for by the prodigious numbers of the small puffballs.

I have seen hundreds of *Lycoperdons* mantling a small area of the woodland floor, crowded together on a pile of sawdust, or covering a stump or log like a multitude of Christmas-tree ornaments. One of these species, the gemmed puffball (*Lycoperdon perlatum*) is so beautiful close up that it reminds me of the delicate eggs fashioned by Carl Fabergé in the nineteenth and early part of the twentieth centuries for the Russian court. The "gems" are actually very tiny cone- or pyramid-shaped spines that dot the white surface of the mushroom like goose bumps (Figure 23). The spines break or rub off easily, leaving smooth spots or scars. The pear-shaped puffballs are 1 to 3 inches high and are white when young, turning a dull tan in age.

The gemmed puffballs, sometimes called devil's snuffbox, grow singly or in great numbers in woodlands. They may be found on rich soil, leafy duff, rotting wood, and other woody debris such as sawdust. The interior of the mushroom is white at first, changing to yellowish to olive brown. The gemmed puffball is one of our most common puffballs and is widely distributed throughout the United States and the rest of the world. It fruits in late summer and fall.

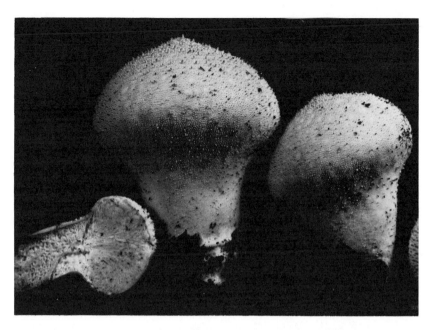

FIGURE 23. *Gemmed puffball* (Lycoperdon perlatum). *The interior of the cut puffball on the left has already begun to darken, so it should not be eaten.*

Another *Lycoperdon*, the pear-shaped puffball (*Lycoperdon pyriforme*) is also a woodland species. It grows on logs and stumps (Color Plate 19). Hundreds of pear-shaped puffballs often cover a stump. I once saw a 15-foot-long slab of bark that was so densely mantled with tan *Lycoperdon pyriforme* that the bark looked like a long tray full of food. This brown mushroom is most common in late summer and fall.

Many years ago, British agricultural scientist P. H. Gregory became intrigued with the *Lycoperdons*, not from a gastronomic viewpoint, but rather as a scientist. Gregory wanted to know more about how spores are released into the air from these small puffballs. He knew that in larger puffballs, spores are disseminated when the outer surface cracks and peels away. Air currents or raindrops scoring a direct hit on an exposed large puffball then send the spores on their way. In smaller puffballs, however, the surface does not crack open. Instead, a tiny hole forms at the top. Dr.

Gregory wondered whether or not the gentle pressure of a raindrop or a gust of wind was sufficient to force the many spores through the tiny opening. The British scientist found the answer after conducting a series of experiments during World War II on the gemmed puffball. In his first experiment at the Rothamsted Experimental Station, Gregory placed the small puffball in a wind tunnel. When winds of ordinary velocity were blown across the puffball's surface, they were not very effective in releasing the spores. Perhaps, Gregory thought, animals such as squirrels, skunks, or chipmunks were spreading the spores of the mushroom when they stepped on the puffballs. However, empty puffballs were found in some areas of England where the footfall of animals could not account for the spore discharge.

Raindrop pressure seemed to be the only possibility left. In an experiment approximating the Chinese water torture technique, Gregory placed a water pipette over a mature gemmed puffball. Periodically, drops of water descended on the puffball. High-speed photography recorded the impact of each drop of water on the puffball's surface. After studying many impacts, Gregory found that raindrops did indeed trigger the release of the puffball's spores. High-speed photographs captured the instant that a drop flattened the papery top of the puffball, sending a tiny cloud of spores about 1 inch into the air.

Excited by this discovery, Gregory carried out his experiment during a normal rainfall to see if he could confirm his laboratory observations. He did. In an article in the *British Mycological Society Transactions* journal in the 1940s, Gregory recalled that the puffball "mechanism was also operated by raindrops under natural conditions." A fine, misty rain didn't produce a puff, noted Gregory, "but thunder rain was excellent." However, even during the fine rain, large drops that collected on the leaves of trees did fall and make "the puffball smoke, as though on fire." Gregory estimated that in an area with an average rainfall of about 40 inches (such as in New England), one large gemmed puffball would be triggered more than 250,000 times by raindrops.

The method of spore dispersal is not the only feature of puffballs that has intrigued scientists. There is the possibility that puffballs may contain a substance that may inhibit cancer. As with many discoveries in science, this finding was uncovered in a roundabout way. E. H. Lucas, a botanist at Michigan State University, was visiting a tiny mountain village near the Bavarian border when he learned that lumberjacks in that area believed that cancer could be prevented by eating a certain type of mushroom, the delicious king bolete (*Boletus edulis*). When Lucas returned to the States, he obtained some of these mushrooms, dried them, mixed them with water, and sent them to the Sloan-Kettering Institute for Cancer Research. Although the extract made from this mushroom was found to be very effective in inhibiting cancerous tumors in mice, Lucas had trouble growing these mushrooms in the laboratory. The mycelium also failed to produce the tumor-inhibitor in the lab. When Lucas tested other mushrooms for cancer-fighting substances, he discovered a very strong tumor-retarding substance in the giant puffball. Lucas remembered other claims that skin cancer could be retarded by spores of puffballs. After further research, a tumor inhibitor was found in the cup-shaped puffball, the brain puffball, and another puffball, *Calvatia bovista*.

The antitumor substance was finally extracted and purified from the giant puffball (*Calvatia gigantea*) and called *calvacin*. Calvacin was then tested against a broad spectrum of cancers in rats, mice, and hamsters. According to a report in *Science Magazine* (December 23, 1960) by J. F. Roland, Lucas, and ten other scientists, calvacin "was found to possess antitumor activity against 14 of 24 various mouse, rat, and hamster tumors." The cancers ranged from those of the skin to those of the lung, bladder, and mammary glands. "This is considered to be a rather broad spectrum type tumor-inhibiting substance," stressed Everett S. Beneke, in his presidential address, "Calvatia, Calvacin, and Cancer," to the 1962 annual meeting of the Mycological Society of America. To obtain more calvacin for toxicity tests and for possible human tests, a total of 1,500 pounds of *Calvatia gigantea* was frozen and shipped to Armour and Company in Chicago for the extraction and purification of calvacin. Approximately 1 pound of purified calvacin was obtained from this huge pile of puffballs. Unfortunately, when calvacin was tested in dogs and monkeys, an apparent allergic reaction was noted in these animals. When the drug was tried on seven human patients with a variety of cancers, the study had to be stopped because calvacin at high dosages turned out to have a toxic effect on muscles, including the heart muscle.

The possible medical benefits of puffballs does not stop with the calvacin experiments. The therapeutic qualities of these large mushrooms have been recognized for centuries. Medical uses of puffballs have been recorded among Asians, Europeans, and North Americans. Such different groups as gypsies in France, villagers in Great Britain, eighteenth- and nineteenth-century European surgeons, and the American Indian have used puffballs to lessen the effects of or to cure various ailments. Perhaps the most widespread application of puffballs was to control bleeding. In the eighteenth century, barbers who also doubled as surgeons used dried spongy puffballs to stop bleeding during and after operations in Great Britain and France. In books such as Gooch's *Treatment of Wounds* (1767), puffballs were recommended as a styptic after amputations. Puffballs were also used as surgical dressings before the advent of antiseptic bandages. As recently as 1910, a medical book by Whitla, *Pharmacy, Materia Medica, and Therapeutics,* recommended the giant puffball as "a soft and comfortable surgical dressing." The book added that "the dusty powder is a powerful haemostat" (substance used to stop bleeding). Puffballs were even used during surgical operations to help anesthetize patients. Fumes given off by the larger puffballs supposedly had properties resembling those of chloroform.

In 1916, a British mycologist reported that puffballs were still being used in some rural areas of Great Britain as a styptic. The dried puffballs were kept as a household remedy in farmhouses and cottages of West Sussex, England, but the mycologist ruefully noted that the custom was rapidly dying out.

Although the North American Indians also used puffballs as a styptic or as a dressing for wounds, many groups of Indians savored these fungi as food. The Pueblo Indians of the Southwest used to gather large numbers of these mushrooms when summer rains wetted the parched earth. They ate some of the puffballs and dried the rest for winter. Puffballs were also a favorite among the Iroquois of the Northeast. Arthur C. Parker, an anthropologist who studied the eating habits of Iroquois at the beginning of this century, told of a simple puffball recipe favored by a tribesman. "Puffballs," wrote Parker in the New York State Museum *Bulletin* in 1910, "were peeled and sliced . . . and fried entire in grease, sunflower, or bear oil." Sometimes deer tallow was used as a substitute.

A puffball has a very subtle taste. To retain the mushroom's original flavor, you should sauté small pieces in butter or margarine. Before sautéing, remove the skin if it is tough.

Puffball slices may also be dipped in batter and deep fried. The mushroom can also be prepared by dipping slices into a mixture of egg, cracker crumbs, and a few herbs, and then frying the puffball slices is butter. My favorite preparation is to stack the fried slices with a layer of sour cream and chives between each slice. Puffballs can also be eaten raw. They can be cut into small cubes, placed on a salad of mixed greens, with the salad dressing being added just before serving.

15 Giant Puffball

EDIBLE, VERY GOOD

Calvatia gigantea
("bald" "gigantic")

COMMON NAMES

Giant puffball, cream puff, devil's snuffbox.

WHAT IT LOOKS LIKE

Fruiting Body: large, nearly round; 8 to 20 inches or more across; outer skin smooth like kid gloves or fine felt; white when young, turning to light gray to yellow or olive when old; outer skin later cracks with age. *Inside:* white like cream cheese when young and edible, becomes yellowish to olive in age as the spores ripen. Thick "root" attached to base.

KEY FEATURES

If you find a large, white, round puffball with a smooth kid-glove surface, you have a giant puffball. Often weighs several pounds.

WHERE FOUND

Occurs alone or in groups of several along edges of meadows, in low, wet areas, along small streams or drainage ditches. Prefers low, rich, wet humus or soil. Widely distributed throughout eastern and central North America.

WHEN

Late summer and on into fall.

16 Western Giant Puffball   EDIBLE, VERY GOOD

Calvatia booniana
("bald" "Boone")

COMMON NAMES

Western giant puffball, giant puffball.

WHAT IT LOOKS LIKE

Fruiting Body: large, slightly flattened, egg-shaped puffball a foot high and up to 2 feet across; outer skin rough and cracked; scaly surface has deep cracks in between the scales when mature; dull white to light tan or buff color. *Inside:* white like cream cheese, later becomes olive brown. Thick root at base.

KEY FEATURES

Similar to the giant white puffball (*Calvatia gigantea*) but has rougher cracked surface.

WHERE FOUND

Grows individually or in twos or threes in the dry open areas of the West. Despite the arid conditions, this mushroom attains a huge size. Look for it under sagebrush, around old corrals, and arid habitats.

WHEN

Late spring and in summer.

17 Cup-shaped Puffball EDIBLE, VERY GOOD

Calvatia cyathiformis
("bald" "cup-shaped")

COMMON NAMES

Cup-shaped puffball, cream puff, pasture puffball, prairie mushroom, devil's snuffbox.

WHAT IT LOOKS LIKE

Fruiting Body: 3 to 6 inches across; has egg-shaped top resting on a thick base; looks like a loaf of bread; outer skin smooth like felt; whitish to pinkish tan to brown; fine cracks lighter in color than rest of surface soon appear; partly wrinkled on sides where top merges with thick base. *Inside:* white like cream cheese (see Color Plate 17B) then yellow to an attractive purple brown.

KEY FEATURES

There are other large puffballs that have a similar size and shape, such as the brain puffball (*Calvatia craniformis*), but all are edible when the interior is white.

WHERE FOUND

Found throughout most of the United States. Fruits on lawns, meadows, pastures, and other open, grassy areas from the East Coast westward to the prairies and into near-desert regions. Forms fairy rings often of huge size. A very common puffball.

WHEN

Late summer and fall after heavy rains.

18 Common Scleroderma   Poisonous

Scleroderma aurantium
("hard skin" "orange")

COMMON NAMES

Earthballs, common scleroderma.

WHAT IT LOOKS LIKE

Fruiting body: 1 to 5 inches across; round to almost kidney-shaped; outer skin tough, thick, yellow-brown; conelike warts on surface; fungus hard as a potato. *Inside:* dull white, quickly becoming purplish black from the center outward; nearly black when mature, surrounded by thick, white outer skin.

KEY FEATURES

The tough outer warty skin, a fungus so hard that you can barely dent it with your finger, and an interior that becomes purple to black so soon that when you break this scleroderma open, it probably will have already turned this color.

WHERE FOUND

The most common of the hard-skinned puffballs. Grows around old stumps, on very rotten logs, in woodlands in northern, eastern, and central North America.

WHEN

Late summer and fall.

19 Pear-shaped Puffball

EDIBLE, GOOD

Lycoperdon pyriforme
("to send forth air" "pear shape")

COMMON NAMES
Pear-shaped puffball, puffball.

WHAT IT LOOKS LIKE
Fruiting Body: small, pear-shaped puffball, about ¾ to nearly 2 inches high, ½ to 1 inch across; skin smooth, sometimes finely cracked or rougher; very pale tan (when in shade) to rusty brown (when exposed to sunlight); strong white threads attached to base so that when one puffball is pulled from a rotten log others attached to the threads often come along (like Christmas-tree lights on a cord). *Inside:* white like cream cheese; becomes yellowish to olive brown.

KEY FEATURES
Clusters of brown, upside-down "pears" (puffballs) growing on rotten wood.

WHERE FOUND
Forms large scattered to crowded clusters on rotten logs, stumps, sawdust piles, and at the base of stumps. Common and widely distributed. Old, papery remains of the puffball last on through the winter and into the next season.

WHEN
Most common late summer and fall.

Fall

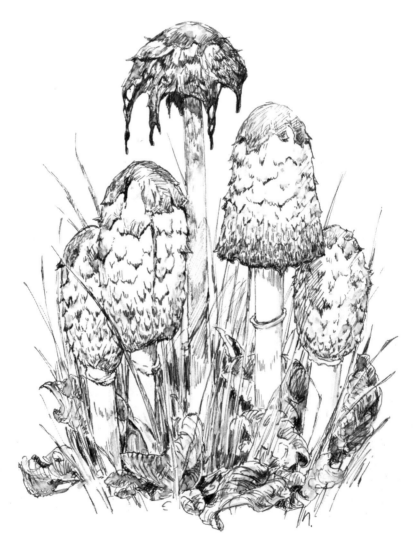

Fall is World Series time for mushrooms, the best collecting
season for many edible wild mushrooms. The largest number of
mushrooms of the entire year will appear during this season. An
infusion of new edible mushrooms will join the many edible mushrooms of late summer; puffballs, meadow mushrooms, and teeth
fungi will continue to fruit into early fall. Fall also means collecting
one of the finest-tasting mushrooms—the king bolete (*Boletus*

edulis), the perfect fall counterpoint to the supreme edible spring species, the morel.

Mushrooming in early September, at least for boletes, means heading for the evergreen forest instead of the deciduous woods and open areas of lawns, fields, and meadows that were frequented during the summer. Although there was a fruiting of summer boletes, they were too often riddled by insects. Early fall is the bolete season for beginners because at that time the cold weather has decimated the population of insect pests and bolete picking is most fruitful. The king bolete (*Boletus edulis*) is found in evergreen forests and in woodlands containing a mixture of evergreens and hardwoods. In the white pines, large fruitings of the painted bolete (*Suillus pictus*) and the granulated bolete (*Suillus granulatus*) carpet the floor of brown needles. In the evergreen forests of the Rocky Mountains and the Pacific Northwest, the beautiful, admirable bolete (*Boletus mirabilis*) grows on rotting logs or stumps, while another attractive, more widespread bolete, the orange bolete (*Leccinum aurantiacum*), is equally at home in evergreen as well as in deciduous woods.

Boletes shouldn't, and don't, monopolize the fall collector's time. In the fall when politicians are out on the stump, so too are many edible fungi. The oyster mushroom and the lilac-spored mushroom (*Pleurotus ostreatus* and *Pleurotus sapidus*) grow on stumps as well as on logs and trees. The cauliflower fungus (*Sparassis radicata*), though sometimes found on a stump, usually grows not too far from a tree because it parasitizes the tree's roots; and the hen of the woods (*Polyporus frondosus*), another edible fungus, is also found around stumps and roots of trees. Other wood-inhabiting fungi such as the brick caps and various polypores are also common in this season.

Meanwhile, on lawns, in hard-packed areas by tennis courts, and along roadsides another edible fall mushroom, the shaggy-mane (*Coprinus comatus*), has joined the puffballs and meadow mushrooms. The shaggy-mane can be collected well into the fall season, after the leaves have dropped from the trees.

When the cold November nights cause temperatures to plummet below freezing, it's time for most mushroomers to call it a season and head indoors.

Bolete

(*Boletus, Suillus,* and *Leccinum*)

KING BOLETE (*Boletus edulis*)
GRANULATED BOLETE (*Suillus granulatus*)
PAINTED BOLETE (*Suillus pictus*)
ADMIRABLE BOLETE (*Boletus mirabilis*)
ORANGE BOLETE (*Leccinum aurantiacum*)
BIRCH BOLETE (*Leccinum scabrum*)

The king bolete belongs to a group of fungi known as boletes. The word comes from the Greek word *bolos*, a "clod," apparently because the mushrooms come up like clods in the woodland. The king bolete is also known as cèpe, steinpilz, porcino, prawdziwy grzyb, and a host of other names throughout the world. Praise has been accorded this famous mushroom for centuries. In Eastern Europe, special trains transport urbanites into the hinterlands each fall to search for this edible bolete. In southern France, the French and the Italians were on the verge of a miniwar when the French discovered that many Italians had gone over the border to collect the bolete in France's woods. In the United States, gourmets, unaware that this famous mushroom grows in their own woodlands, flock to specialty food shops to buy dried boletes at $30 a pound.

Why is there such a furor over this mushroom? To non-mushroom lovers, the king bolete certainly does not look special. The mushroom has a large, round, brown cap that looks like a hamburger bun (Figure 24). Underneath the cap, where you

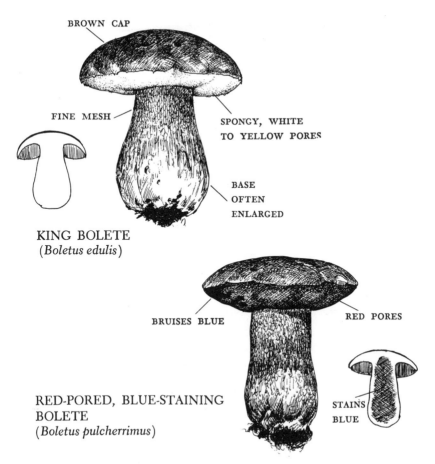

BROWN CAP

FINE MESH

SPONGY, WHITE
TO YELLOW PORES

BASE
OFTEN
ENLARGED

KING BOLETE
(*Boletus edulis*)

BRUISES BLUE

RED PORES

RED-PORED, BLUE-STAINING
BOLETE
(*Boletus pulcherrimus*)

STAINS
BLUE

FIGURE 24. *Key features of a king bolete* (Boletus edulis) *and a red-pored blue-staining bolete* (Boletus pulcherrimus).

would expect the gills to be found, is a spongy layer peppered with hundreds of tiny holes. The bolete's stem, adorned partly or entirely with a fine white mesh, tapers outward like a club or has a bulblike base. The mushroom is most often found under pine and other evergreen trees.

When you taste the king bolete, you quickly learn why the adulation for this mushroom is warranted. With the possible— and I stress the word *possible*—exception of the morel, the king bolete to me is the finest-tasting mushroom known to humankind. Few tastes are as elegant as a king bolete that has been briefly sautéed in butter only a few hours after it has been picked. The taste is a combination of sweetness and nuttiness that is truly distinctive; its texture is crunchy.

The boletes resemble a gilled mushroom in that they have a cap and a stipe, but the spongy layer underneath the cap separates the boletes from the agarics (gilled mushrooms). Another group of mushrooms, the polypores, also have tiny holes (pores), but they grow on wood, whereas nearly all boletes grow on the ground. Polypores are also usually tough to woody and generally do not have a stem.

The bolete pores in the spongy layer are the openings of tiny tubes that crowd together along the bottom of the cap. If the cap were cut in half down toward the stalk, a layer of many parallel tubes open only at the bottom (the pores) would be seen lining the underside of the fleshy cap (see the small drawing in Figure 24). In most boletes, this tube layer separates very easily from the cap's tissue.

The spores of the bolete form along the inside walls of the tubes. After the spores mature, they are forcibly discharged from the tube walls. They fall through a tube and out into the air where winds carry the spores to a new site.

The boletes include some of the best edible mushrooms. They are also one of the safest groups of mushrooms to eat provided a few simple rules are observed. Avoid all boletes that (1) have red pores, (2) stain blue, and (3) have a bitter taste. If you follow these rules, a pleasant repast of boletes can be enjoyed many times throughout the fall season.

(1) *Avoid red pore boletes* (Figure 24 and Color Plate 26). Some boletes with red pores, though not deadly, may cause vomiting, cramps, or diarrhea. Even though there are boletes with red pores that are edible, beginners should avoid all red-pore boletes because of the presence of some poisonous species. The red-pore boletes can be easily separated from the edible boletes because the pore color stands out like a red flag, warning collectors to stay away.

(2) *Boletes that stain blue upon handling should also be avoided.* In these boletes, a blue color may appear if the mushroom is cut open, touched, or handled in any way. The amount

and rapidity of the color change depends on the species. The bluing may be rapid or slow. It may be confined only to an area of the pore surface that has been scratched or pushed in with a finger. In other species, the bluing may extend through the entire flesh when the mushroom is cut open with a knife. It may also appear just by touching the stem or cap surface. Color Plate 26 dramatically illustrates what happens when you scratch the stem and poke the pore surface of the red-pored *Boletus subvelutipes*. The damaged areas quickly turn an intense blue and then change to a darker blue-black.

The bluing reaction is a chemical change similar to that occurring in certain fruits when they are cut open. The surface becomes oxidized when exposed to the air, just as the flesh of an apple oxidizes and turns brown when the fruit is cut open. Two chemicals in boletes play an important role in the bluing of the mushroom tissue. They are called *boletol* and *laccase*. Normally, these chemicals are found separately in the tissue. However, when the tissues are bruised or cut open, the chemicals merge and react in the presence of oxygen in the air. The laccase and the oxygen cause the boletol to turn blue. If only a little laccase is present, the color change is slight. If the mushroom contains more laccase, the bluing becomes deeper in color. Although some people have become ill eating boletes that stain blue, the chemicals that cause the bluing are not to blame. It turns out that other chemicals, still not identified, cause the stomach upsets. In fact, many species of boletes that turn blue are edible and very good. But because *some* bluing species do cause upsets, beginners should avoid all blue-stained boletes.

(3) *Avoid all boletes that taste bitter.* These boletes are not poisonous, simply unpalatable because of their bitter taste. Surprisingly, other mushroom books almost invariably fail to list this criterion with the blue-staining, red-pore characteristics as *general* features to avoid when collecting boletes for the table. One group of boletes (*Tylopilus*) contains several species with a bitter taste. Although the pores of these bitter mushrooms eventually attain a pinkish cast when the pink spores of the mushroom mature and appear at the mouths of the tubes, the spongy underside of these

mushrooms are cream to white at first. At this period, the species may be confused with some nonbitter boletes.

A simple taste test will quickly rule out the bitter boletes. If a small piece of the mushroom cap is placed on the tip of the tongue, the taste buds will quickly indicate that the mushroom is a bitter bolete. In rare cases, people with taste buds that are not especially sensitive to a bitter taste may take somewhat longer to detect the bitterness. Chris Kolej, a bolete devotee in a Connecticut mushroom club to which I belong, says that the bitter taste disappears after the mushroom is dried. Others claim that repeated washings of the bolete will also get rid of the bitter taste. However, it is best to avoid all bitter boletes.

In most parts of the United States, boletes have two main periods of fruiting: summer and fall. In midsummer, after a good rain, the deciduous woodlands occupy center stage for the boletes. The woodland floor under oaks, birches, and other trees may explode with a tremendous variety. Edible boletes along with the blue stainers and red pores proliferate in the humid summer weather. More boletes appear during this period than at any other time of year. Toward the end of summer, the fruiting in the deciduous woodlands fades, and the bolete scene shifts in the fall mainly to the coniferous or evergreen woods. There, the king bolete along with the butterballs (*Suillus*) and other boletes fruit, often in tremendous quantities.

Because of this dual fruiting period, it seemed at first difficult to choose where the bolete section should be placed in the seasonal chronology of this book. The boletes could have been divided into two groups, the summer boletes and the fall boletes with a separate section for each. Adding to the confusion was the fact that the king bolete seemed to straddle both seasons. In many regions, it fruits both in late summer and in the fall. However, some tiny organisms that vie with humans in the pursuit of boletes helped resolve my dilemma. In actual fact, the best time for *picking* boletes is in the fall, when intrusion by insect larvae is at a minimum. Hence the placement of boletes in this season.

During humid summer weather, picking boletes can be a frustrating experience. A collector often races with the insects to see who gets to the boletes first. The insects win most of the time. Sometimes, beautiful specimens are found that seem to have escaped the insect invasion. However, as soon as the mushrooms are cut open, the interiors are found to be riddled with tiny tunnels or holes filled with robust larvae.

The thick, fleshy boletes are choice foods for the insect larvae. The larvae usually enter the mushroom through the base of the stalk and work upward toward the cap. The warmer the weather, the faster they travel. The larvae work so fast that boletes, even at the small button stage, are often overtaken by the insects. Glistening cellophanelike trails on some boletes indicate that slugs also find the boletes delicious. I have had many choice meals from boletes collected during the summer, but the percentage of insect-free mushrooms is usually small. Although some species seem to be less favored and even ignored by insects, the best success rate is obtained in the fall when the cold weather reduces the activity of insects.

The growth habits of boletes greatly simplify the search for these delicious mushrooms. Boletes are primarily mycorrhizal; the mycelia link with the roots of particular trees. Many form unique partnerships only with certain trees; other species are more cosmopolitan, linking with several kinds of trees. The relationship between boletes and trees provides an excellent clue to help you find boletes more easily. For example, when you visit a grove of white pine trees, you can expect to find the painted bolete (*Suillus pictus*) and the granulated bolete (*Suillus granulatus*). Both species form mycorrhizae with white pines. If you find a white birch, look for a gray-brown-capped bolete (*Leccinum scabrum*) with a stem that looks as if it had been charred by a fire. Once, I thought that I had found a rare exception to this bolete's usual mycorrhizal relationship with birches when I spotted a solitary *Leccinum scabrum* in a white pine grove whose needled floor was mantled with dozens of painted and granulated boletes. However, I soon saw a lone birch sapling growing a few feet away from the bolete in a small opening among the pines.

Such a linkage happens repeatedly when a collector is searching for boletes. If you come across a certain bolete, you can often name the tree that is nearby without even looking up. Mushroom collectors, of course, work the other way around. They go to the woodlands where trees with which the boletes are associated grow. Then they look for the particular boletes. Boletes form mycorrhizae with most evergreen trees. Among deciduous trees, boletes form mycorrhizae most often with birch, aspen, oak, and beech.

Another growth habit of boletes is that they fruit in very accessible areas and can be collected with a minimum of effort. "When hunting for boletes, often the easiest technique pays off," say bolete authorities Alexander H. Smith and Harry D. Thiers in their comprehensive book, *The Boletes of Michigan*. Boletes have a habit of fruiting along old roads through the woods, along the edges of wood lots, around isolated trees in old fields and pastures, and along fence rows where there are trees in which the boletes form mycorrhizae. I have often filled up my basket with boletes simply by walking in a grassy area along the edge of a woodland. The boletes were clustered in the grass where the roots of the mycorrhizal trees extended out into the field's soil. Even in the woodlands themselves, boletes fruit most abundantly in accessible spots such as the open, needle-strewn floor under evergreens or in thin deciduous woods.

The boletes in the United States are a diverse group, whose species number in the hundreds. In *The Boletes of Michigan* alone, about two hundred species are listed. Scientists group the boletes according to how the pores are arranged under the cap, by spore color, by the presence of small tufts on the stipe, and other characteristics. This section presents only a sampling of the boletes. These species, however, are among the best-eating, most easily recognized, and most widely collected boletes.

Leading the list, of course, is the king bolete (*Boletus edulis*), which generally forms a mycorrhizal relationship with pines, hemlocks, and other evergreens. (However, one variety also grows under birch and aspen.) To find this bolete, tramp through evergreen stands in a woodland containing a mixture of evergreens and hardwoods or in an area where birch and aspen are found. Look for a chunky bolete (Color Plate 20) with a brown to red-brown cap and a thick, clublike stipe that is partly or entirely covered with a white netting or mesh (reticulation). The white reticulation on the white to pale-brown stem looks like a frosted version of very fine chicken wire mesh that was either wrapped around the entire stem or just around the top part near the mushroom cap.

In the young king bolete, the tube layer underneath the cap is white; it then changes to yellow with a greenish tinge at maturity. The king bolete grows on the ground singly or in clusters of two to five.

The mushroom is aptly named. It is not only kingly in taste but also in size. Occasionally giant 5-pound specimens with caps a foot in diameter are found. Many tall stories about boletes have turned out to be true. Margaret Lewis, the diminutive septuagenarian of the Boston Mycological Club and an avid hiker, recalls struggling down from the higher elevations of the Rockies with a backpack full of many 5-pound *Boletus edulis*. All of the large mushrooms were perfectly edible, in their prime, and did not have a trace of insect infestation. However, the ordinary collector cannot expect to find such specimens on every occasion. The king boletes most often seen are usually smaller, though still a good size, with caps about 3 to 6 inches in diameter.

You should probably start looking for the king bolete in late summer after a heavy rain. In most parts of the country, the fruiting occurs from late August and into fall. The fruiting pattern of *Boletus edulis* seems to be erratic. This prima donna of the mushroom world may appear in great numbers in some years, with only a few in other years. Weather conditions, of course, are a critical factor, although the mushroom may be abundant in what seems to be a relatively dry season.

Several varieties of mushrooms are grouped under the name *Boletus edulis*. All have the typical characteristics of a chunky bolete with white, netlike reticulations on the stem, a hamburger-bun-shaped cap, and a white to yellow pore surface. The differences among the varieties are relatively minor. One variety, for example, has a rosy-tan color on the cap instead of a brown bun color. Another variety grows under birch and aspen. This variety was the one I picked with my parents when I was a young boy. Even though we collected several kinds of boletes, this one was called *borowik* or *prawdziwy*, which in Polish meant "the best" in taste. It was. However, regardless of the variety of *Boletus edulis* found, all are equally delicious.

There is one inedible bolete that beginners in the central and eastern part of the United States may confuse with the king bolete. It's the pink-spored bitter bolete (*Tylopilus felleus*). Though not poisonous, this mushroom has an extremely bitter taste. Like the king bolete, the bitter bolete grows under evergreens. It is usually found around old hemlock stumps in the summer and fall. This mushroom also has a brown cap and a stalk with reticulations. However, several key characteristics will immediately separate the two species (Color Plates 20 and 21). The reticulation on the stalk is dark brown, not white; the taste is very bitter (one bite is sufficient), and the pore surface of a mature bitter bolete is pink, not white or yellow. Young specimens of the bitter bolete at first have a white to cream pore surface, as in young king boletes, but the dark brown reticulation and the bitter taste are enough to distinguish this bolete from *Boletus edulis*. Fortunately, mushroom collectors who do not live in the central or eastern part of the United States don't have to worry about these distinctions because the bitter bolete (*Tylopilus felleus*) is known to grow only in those regions.

Several other delicious boletes are found under evergreens. They include the granulated bolete, the painted bolete, and the admirable bolete. The first is found under pines throughout most of the United States, the second under white pine, and the third species, which is most common in the Pacific Northwest and Rocky Mountain states, has the unusual distinction of being one of the few boletes that grows *on* rotten logs or stumps as well as in the soil.

The granulated bolete (*Suillus granulatus*) has many common names, including butterball and old sticky bun. The latter name was appended to this mushroom because of the sticky coating of its cap. When this mushroom pushes up through the needled mat, some of the pine needles may stick to the cap. The stickiness is especially evident when the cap is wet. When preparing this mushroom to eat, the sticky coating can be wiped off or removed by

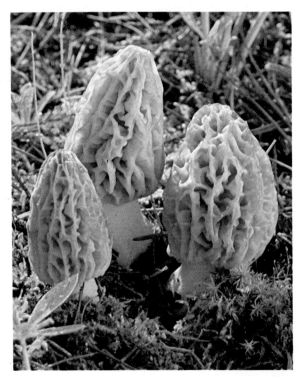

1. Common morel
(Morchella esculenta)

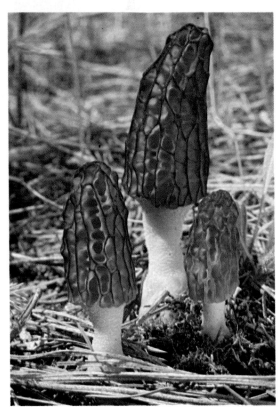

2. Black morel
(Morchella angusticeps)

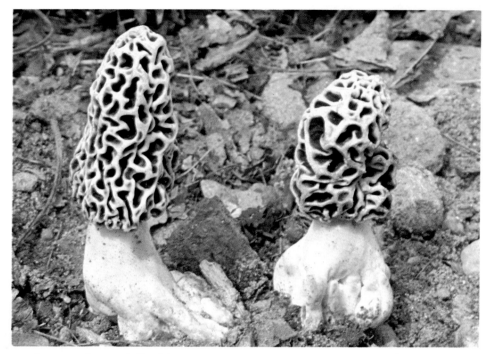

3. White morel *(Morchella deliciosa)*

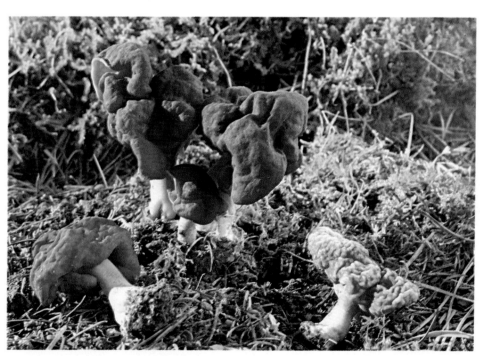

4. False morel *(Gyromitra esculenta)*   Poisonous

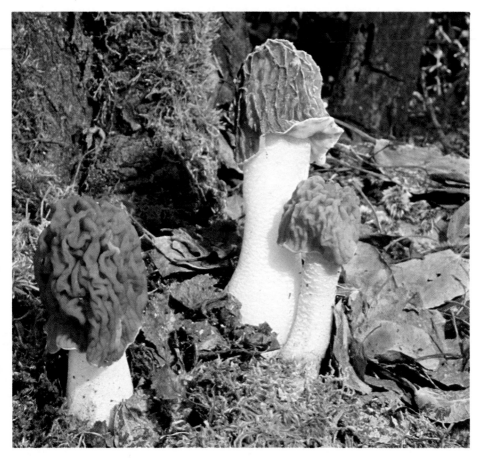

5. Early morel *(Verpa bohemica)* POISONOUS

A B

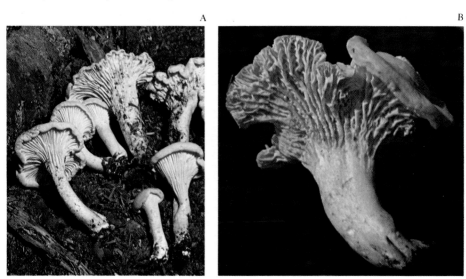

6. Golden chanterelle *(Cantharellus cibarius)*

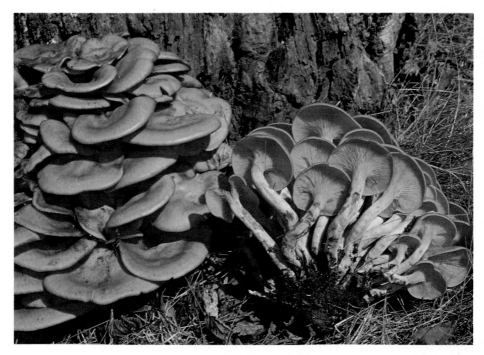

7. Jack-o'-lantern fungus *(Omphalotus illudens)*   POISONOUS

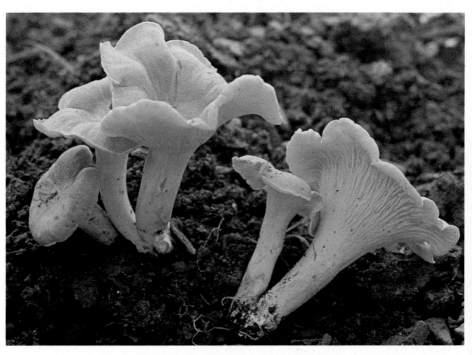

8. Gill-less chanterelle *(Craterellus cantharellus)*

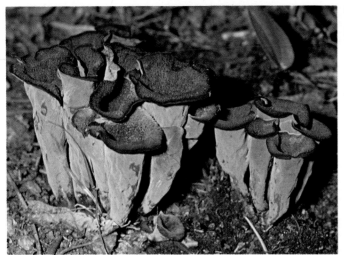

9. Horn of plenty
(*Craterellus cornucopioides*)

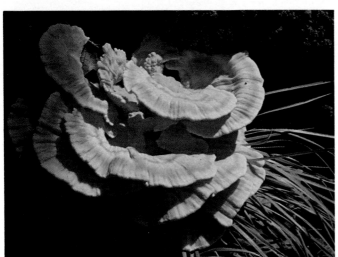

10. Sulphur shelf
mushroom
(*Polyporus sulphureus*)

A. Top

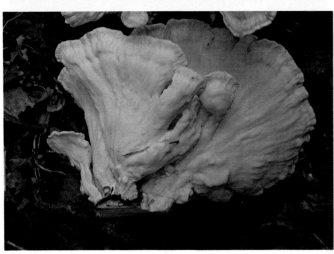

B. Underside

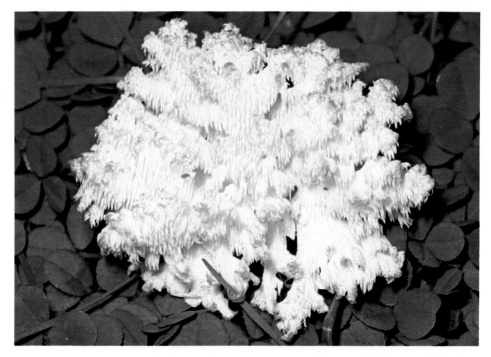

11. Coral hydnum *(Hericium coralloides)*

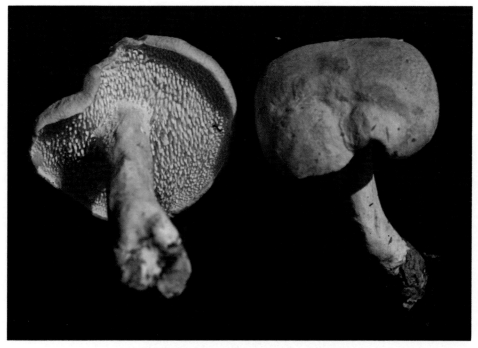

12. Hedgehog mushroom *(Dentinum repandum)*

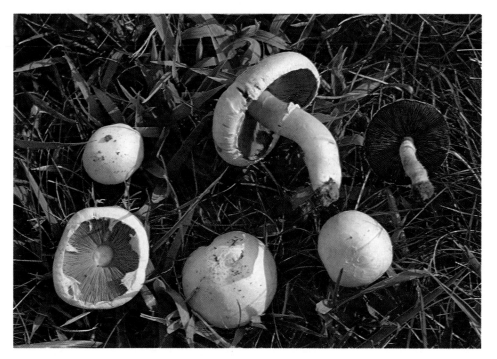

13. Meadow mushroom *(Agaricus campestris)*

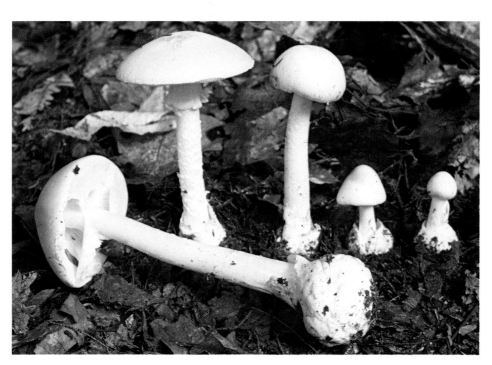

14. Destroying angel *(Amanita virosa)* POISONOUS

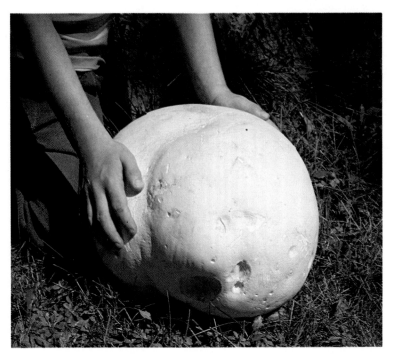

15. Giant puffball *(Calvatia gigantea)*

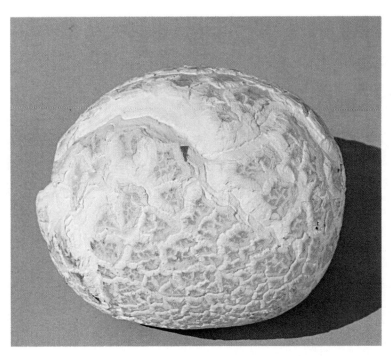

16. Western giant puffball *(Calvatia booniana)*

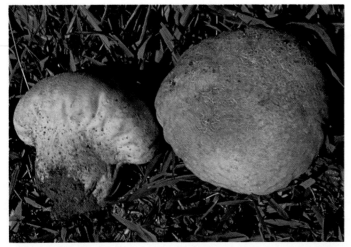

17. Cup-shaped puffball
(Calvatia cyathiformis)

A. Outside

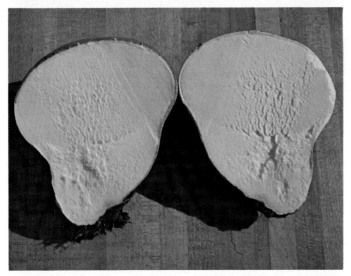

B. Cross Section

18. Common scleroderma
(Scleroderma aurantium)

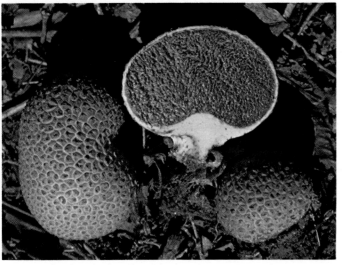

POISONOUS

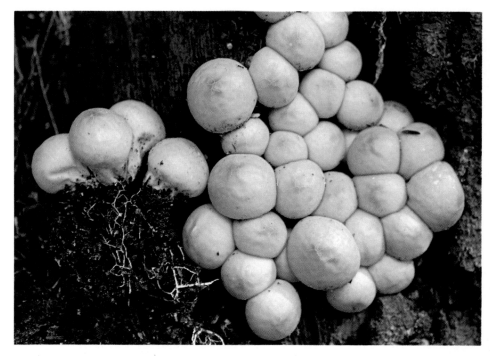

19. Pear-shaped puffball *(Lycoperdon pyriforme)*

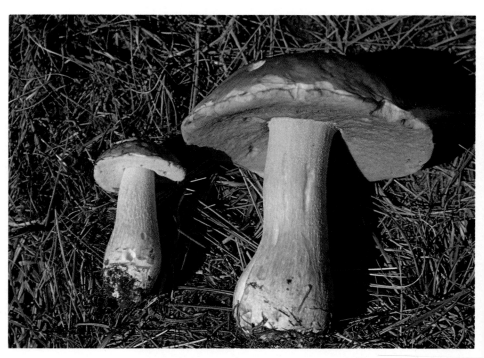

20. King bolete *(Boletus edulis)*

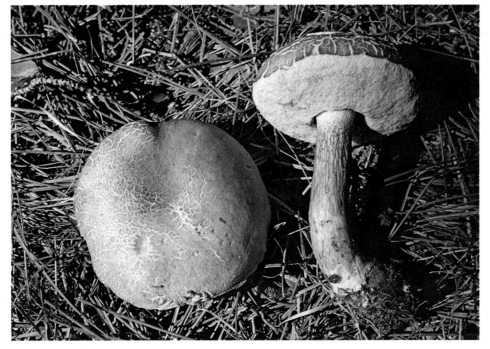

21. Bitter bolete *(Tylopilus felleus)*   INEDIBLE

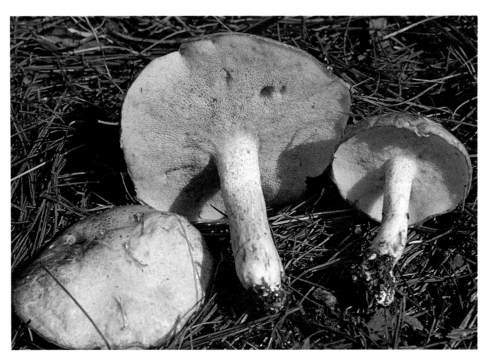

22. Granulated bolete *(Suillus granulatus)*

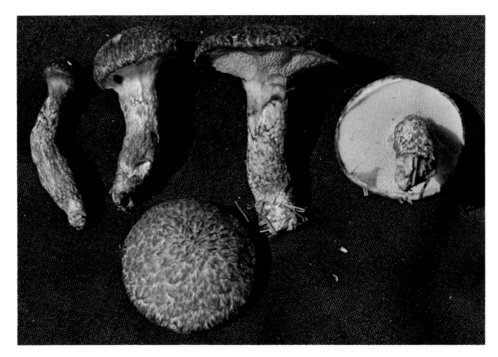

23. Painted bolete *(Suillus pictus)*

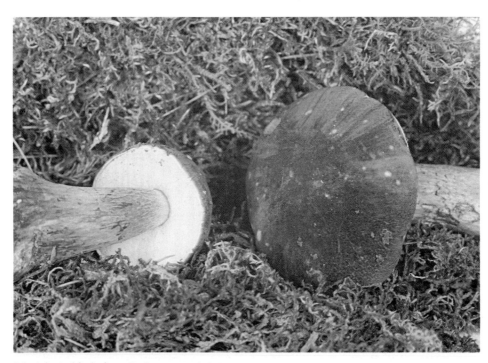

24. Admirable bolete *(Boletus mirabilis)*

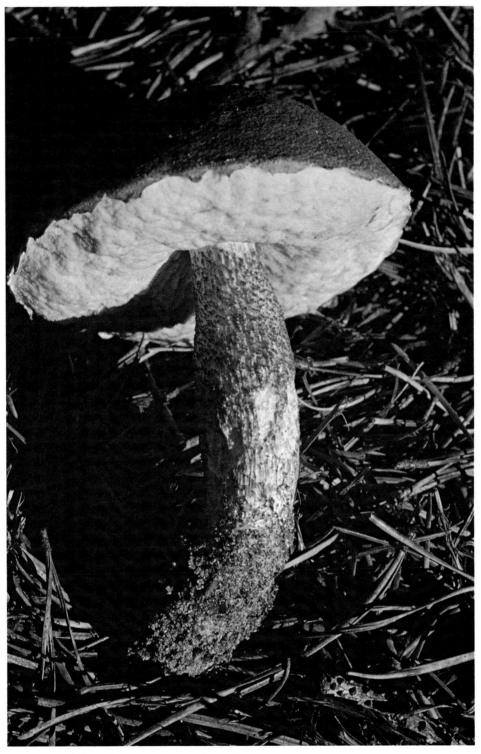

25. Orange bolete (*Leccinum aurantiacum*)

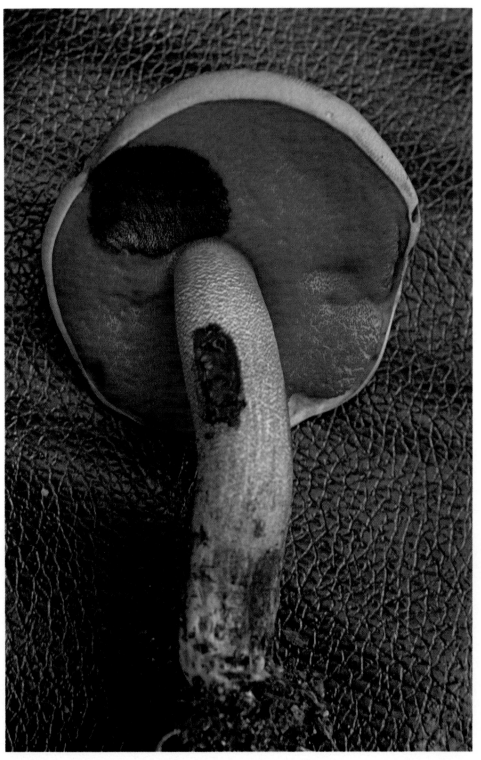

26. Red-pored blue-staining bolete

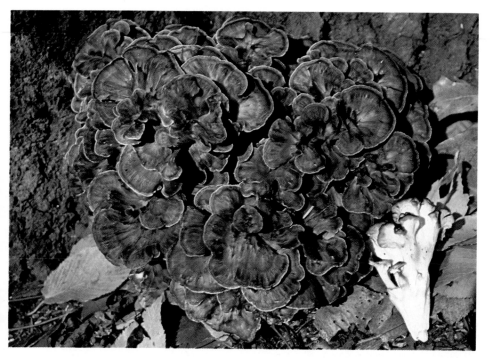

27. Hen of the woods (*Polyporus frondosus*)

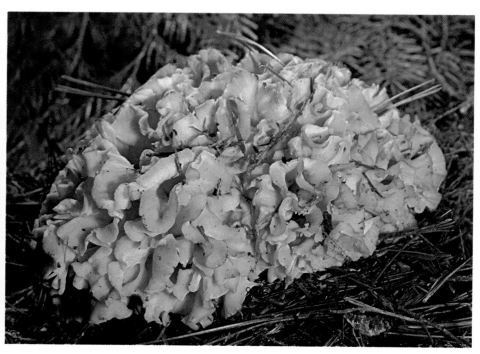

28. Cauliflower fungus (*Sparassis radicata*)

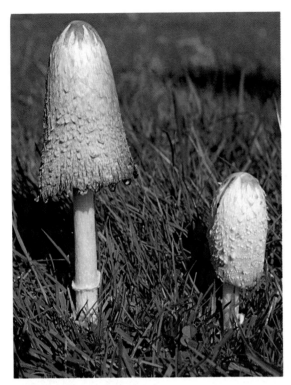

29. Shaggy-mane
(Coprinus comatus)

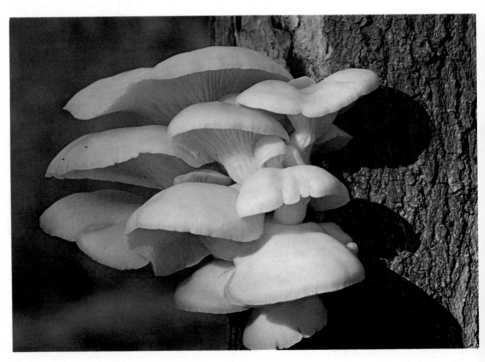

30. Lilac-spored mushroom *(Pleurotus sapidus)*

peeling the *cuticle*, the outside covering of the mushroom. The cap is generally pale brown and is about 2 to 6 inches in diameter. A key characteristic of the granulated bolete is the tiny tan to rosy-brown dots that speckle the whitish stalk (Color Plate 22). The stalk looks as if it were sprinkled with paprika or, when examined under a hand lens, as if it were covered with tiny blobs of dried paint. The tube layer of the graulated bolete is white during the button stage, turning to pale yellow in age.

The granulated bolete is found under various species of pines; it is especially abundant under eastern white pine, those beautiful, soft, blue-green pagodalike evergreens native to the eastern part of the United States and grown as ornamental trees in other regions. These pines have long needles that grow in clusters of five. I start looking for the granulated bolete in September, when the katydid stridulations start winding down with the first cool nights, when the first tufts of goldenrod blossoms appear, and after a heavy rain has soaked the spongy needled soil beneath the pines. I visit a stand of wild white pines, or a lawn, country club grounds, park, or reservoir where white pines have been planted. Once a granulated bolete site has been discovered, a person can return each fall after a rain to find the mushroom. Sometimes one white pine will yield enough boletes for a meal. I once saw a few dozen granulated boletes underneath a white pine that grew alone on a greensward near a highway exit ramp. Even though no other pines were nearby, at one time some peripatetic spores of this bolete found conditions ripe for growth in the isolated island of soil beneath the pine. (A word of caution: If you find boletes or any other edible mushroom near a busy highway, don't pick them. Emissions from passing autos may contaminate the mushrooms.)

Another white-pine inhabitant is the beautiful painted bolete (*Suillus pictus*). This red bolete with the yellow pores does look as if it would be a perfect subject for an artist to paint (Color Plate 23). In the button stage, this mushroom has a tiny pointed cap that has a rich burgundy color. As the mushroom becomes older, the cap expands, and the clumps of hairy reddish scales that gave the mushroom its burgundy hue separate, revealing areas of underlying yellow. At this stage, the cap surface resembles the kind of red brocaded walls seen in some fine restaurants. During its youth, the painted bolete also has a cottony veil that bridges the rim of the cap and the long, red-streaked stalk. When the mushroom cap expands, the veil separates, leaving part of it hanging from the edge of the cap like a miniskirt with the rest forming a ring on the stalk.

The mushroom grows about 5 inches high. The openings of the yellow pores are so large that you can readily see inside the pores. The painted bolete, a distinctive inhabitant of the white pines, is one of my favorite edible mushrooms.

A choice bolete that grows in the evergreen forests of the Rocky Mountains and the Pacific Northwest is the western contender for a beauty prize among the boletes. This mushroom is the admirable bolete (*Boletus mirabilis*). With its velvety maroon-brown cap and bright sulphur-yellow pores, it also has the unusual characteristic of growing on rotten hemlock logs or stumps as well as in the soil (Color Plate 24). The cap is perched on a long, brown stalk that is sometimes reticulated, as with the king bolete. However, this feature is not reliable; in some seasons, the reticulation is not present. The lush-looking cap is 3 to 6 inches wide; the stipe 6 inches long. The flesh is firm and has an excellent, delicate flavor.

Although insects do not attack the admirable bolete as readily as other boletes, white mold sometimes forms on the mushroom. Discard any of the mushrooms that carry this mold.

As mentioned earlier, one variety of *Boletus edulis* grows under birch and aspen trees. There is also another group of boletes that grow in the fall under deciduous trees as well as under evergreens. Mycologists call this group *Leccinum*, yet a more popular name could be the sooty (or singed) boletes because the white stalks look as if they had been singed by a forest fire. Upon closer examination, the sooty particles of these mushrooms turn out to be tiny dark-brown to black tufts that rise from the stalks. These hairy tufts are minute, elongated cells that have clustered together. If these tufts were hard, the stalks would make a good rasp.

The *Leccinum* is a tall robust mushroom. Its stalk is long (3 to 7 inches) and the cap is almost always shaped like a hamburger bun. Its pincushion tube layer is generally some shade of yellow to yellow brown.

"All of the species of *Leccinum* are edible," according to Orson K. Miller, Jr., in his encyclopedic *Mushrooms of North America.* In Michigan, which has an unusually large number of *Leccinums*, all of the many species that have been eaten were found to be edible. If any poisonous species of *Leccinum* occur, say Alexander H. Smith and Harry D. Thiers in *The Boletes of Michigan*, we should have learned about them by now. Even so, when sampling a *Leccinum* (or any other mushroom) for the first time, observe the usual precaution of trying only a little bit at first to make sure you do not have any reactions.

The most prized edible among the species of *Leccinum* is the orange bolete (*Leccinum aurantiacum*). This large, robust mushroom has a bright, rusty red to orange-red cap and a large, chunky, white stalk covered with dark brown to blackish tufts (Color Plate 25). This mushroom is found most commonly under aspen and pines. It fruits in fall as well as at the end of summer. Each fall, I find large numbers of these mushrooms under the coastal pitch pines of New England. The huge caps, totally free of insects, are often about the size of pie plates.

When cut, the white flesh of the mushroom changes slowly to gray with reddish overtones. The red is so slight that it can easily be overlooked. As the flesh becomes darker gray, a slight bluish cast can be discerned in the gray. The entire color change may take several minutes to complete. The color change is more rapid and pronounced in the flesh of the stalk than in the cap.

This slight bluing emphasizes the fact that not all blue-staining boletes are poisonous. In fact, once the *Leccinum* group can be recognized, the caution to beginners to avoid blue-staining boletes can be ignored, *but only for the Leccinum.* This exception to the general rule was brought home to me on a visit to my parents. At that time, I had developed a deep interest in mushrooms again after a long hiatus between my youthful days when I used to tag along with my father and my adult years when I went on to pursue other interests. I was, as an adult, in effect beginning all over again. That fall day, with my head full of newly acquired book knowledge about mushrooms, I told my father that you should never eat boletes that stain blue when cut. With a hearty laugh, my father pointed out that he had been eating blue-staining boletes for years and had never become ill. Of course, he had been eating some of the exceptions to the blue-staining rule and one of these exceptions—the orange-capped *Leccinum aurantiacum*—grew among the aspen saplings at the edge of a field behind our house.

The orange bolete tastes very good, although it does not rank as high as the king bolete. Although the orange bolete blackens upon cooking, this color change does not affect the flavor. Many animals, including mice, deer, turtles, and squirrels, like to eat this mushroom and other boletes. Squirrels dry and store boletes in various ways for the winter. In Jamestown, New York, so many boletes were once found festooning dead branches beneath the needled canopy of a red-pine forest that the trees looked as if they were decorated with Christmas-tree candles. Red squirrels had placed the mushrooms on the branches stem side up.

Other species of *Leccinum* are also collected by humans in the fall. They include sooty-stemmed boletes with gray-brown, blackish, or even greenish-white caps. All have the typical dark-brown to black tufts on the stipe; all are safe to eat. These mushrooms form mycorrhizae with birch, aspen, beech, and various evergreens. One such species is the birch bolete (*Leccinum scabrum*), so named because it is found most commonly under birch. Although similar to *Leccinum aurantiacum*, the birch bolete is usually smaller and more slender and has a gray-brown cap. The mushroom, which is also known as the rough-stemmed bolete, is not as tasty as the orange-capped *Leccinum aurantiacum*. Unfortunately, it also is frequently riddled with insect larvae (Figure 25). However, if you collect this mushroom in the cooler temperature of fall, the chances are that these mushrooms will be relatively free of insect damage.

Boletes, whether they be orange, painted, or king boletes, may be prepared in many ways. To the purists, the king bolete's delicious, sweet, nutty taste can best be appreciated by simply sautéing the mushroom in butter. The fewer the ingredients added,

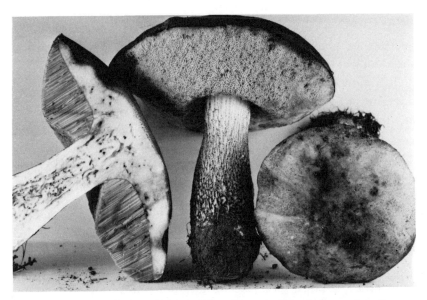

FIGURE 25. *Birch Bolete* (Leccinum scabrum). *The holes and pathways made by insects in the flesh are a common problem, especially in warm weather. The colder weather of fall reduces the intrusions. Note the sooty stem typical of a Leccinum.*

the better. And the purists have an excellent point. However, boletes are also delicious when prepared in other ways. A classic recipe is the French *cèpe provençal*, in which king boletes are sautéed in butter with garlic and parsley. In another classic recipe, *cèpe bordelaise*, the king boletes are sautéed in olive oil with shallots. The word *cèpe*, in French, means "trunk," referring to the chunky stem. Still another favorite is the creamy German white sauce used with boletes, or *steinpilz* ("stone mushroom"). Two of these recipes can be found on page 209.

Boletes are also excellent mushrooms to dry, as the squirrels have discovered. Drying distills the essence of the bolete's flavor. Small buttons may be dried whole, but large caps should be cut into thin slices. Some people dry the mushrooms by putting them in the sun and turning them over periodically. When dried, the mushrooms may be stored in jars or strung together by inserting a thread through the caps and pieces. In some European countries, a string of boletes are hung over a stove to dry. My relatives in southeastern Poland frequently send our family a mushroom necklace of king boletes, a mushroom that grows abundantly in the woods in their region. If sold in gourmet shops in this country, such a choice string of boletes would be worth up to $15. The dried mushrooms, when reconstituted with water or milk, are good in soups, sauces, and casseroles.

The role of a particular food in the culture of a country can be gauged by how often it is singled out in books, paintings, poetry, cooking, and other arts. Boletes and other mushrooms figure prominently in the culture of Eastern European countries. In Russia, children are taught to appreciate mushrooms at an early age, when their parents and *babushka*, or grandmother, read children's poems or stories about boletes. In classic Russian and Polish books, such authors as Boris Pasternak, Tolstoy, and Adam Mickiewicz, a Polish poet, beautifully describe various encounters with boletes and other mushrooms. In *Anna Karenina*, for example, Tolstoy wrote of peasants collecting boletes while simultaneously cutting down grasses with a scythe among the birches, and of children with their governess gathering a whole basketful of birch boletes. In the same book there is even a pleasant, humorous mushroom interlude between the older Sergey Ivanovitch Koznishev, and the beautiful young Varenka, in which Sergey Ivanovitch is trying to summon up courage to ask Varenka to marry him and Varenka, expecting such a proposal, bides her time by walking along the edge of a woodland, collecting mushrooms. Each time Sergey Ivanovitch decides to propose to Varenka, the subject of mushrooms comes up instead. In a tender love scene, Tolstoy wrote:

> He [Sergey Ivanovitch] even said over to himself the words in which he meant to put his offer, but instead of these words, some utterly unexpected reflection that occurred to him made him ask, "What is the difference between the 'birch' mushroom and the 'white' mushroom?" Varenka's lips quivered with emotion as she answered: "In the top part there is scarcely any difference, it's in the stalk."
>
> And as soon as these words were uttered, both he and she felt that it was over, that what was to have been said

would not be said; and their emotion, which had up to then been continually growing more intense, began to subside. "The birch mushroom's stalk suggests a dark man's chin after two days without shaving," said Sergey Ivanovitch, speaking quite calmly now. "Yes, that's true," answered Varenka, smiling, and unconsciously the direction of their walk changed. . . .

The proposal never materialized. The reader with an interest in mushrooms was left with a very good description of the birch *Leccinum* while the reader with a flair for romance was left frustrated. The white mushroom, by the way, was the *Boletus edulis*, and the white referred to the color of the mesh on the light stem.

In Lithuania, now part of the Soviet Union, the people pay homage to boletes in an unusual culinary way. During the Christmas holidays, they prepare mushroom cookies, or *grybai*. These cookies, which look like boletes, are the traditional way of celebrating the role of wild foods in Lithuanian culture.

The mushroom cookie is the "official" Lithuanian Christmas cookie. The cookies have a chocolate-brown cap with a "pore surface" and stem made with a white frosting. Some of the cookies are shaped like the button stage of the mushroom; others are much larger; all are—without question—edible. This Lithuanian tradition of mushroom cookies has been transplanted to American shores. I have seen the mushroom for sale in Lithuanian booths at local ethnic festivals, and I know of persons of Lithuanian descent who still make the cookies.

The Slavic people certainly do not have a monopoly on the ancient tradition of eating boletes. In Italy, for example, the Italians trace their love of porcino, or the king bolete, back to the glories of the Roman Empire. During the zenith of various cultures, mushrooms occupied a lofty position among royalty and other leaders of society. In Egypt, mushrooms could only be eaten by the Pharaohs; such gastronomical gems were not to be wasted on the common people. In France, during the enlightened seventeenth-century reign of King Louis XIV, the discovery that a close relative of the meadow mushroom could be cultivated in gardens triggered a royal interest. Again, mushrooms were grown only for the privileged. During the time of the Roman Empire, when the pleasures of the table were so important, fungi, including boletes, were cherished as "food of the gods." The fungi were considered so valuable that a slave could not be trusted to carry mushrooms to a friend of the slave's owner, because he would certainly eat the fungi along the way, according to the Roman author Martial (A.D. 43–104). "Yet, this same slave," said Martial, "could be trusted with gold or silver to his care." Roman gentlemen were so possessive of their fungi that they personally cooked the fungi—the only cooking these men would condescend to do. The mushrooms would be prepared in special vessels called boletaria, and were eaten with amber knives and silver service. The boletaria could not be used for any purposes other than preparing mushrooms. In an epigram, Martial once bewailed the fallen state of a boletaria when it was used to prepare brussel sprouts instead of fungi.

The most favored mushroom in Rome was, ironically, an edible amanita. The mushroom that was considered *the* "food of the gods" was the orange amanita or Caesar's mushroom (*Amanita caesarea*). This delicious fungus has an orange-yellow cap and a stem that rises out of a white, cuplike base. Caesar's mushroom was the imperial mushroom of Rome. The king bolete was also eaten although the Romans did not consider it as good as the orange amanita. In another epigram, Martial complains that when he was invited to a banquet, Ponticus, a Roman poet, was offered the Caesar's mushroom but he had to be content with the king bolete. At the time this bolete had the ignoble name of *suilli*, which means "hog fungi." This name was given to *Boletus edulis* because the Romans observed that swine were fond of the mushrooms. Recipes for preparing these mushrooms are found in the celebrated Roman cookbook *De Arte Coquinaria*, whose recipes are attributed to the Roman epicure and bon vivant Marcus Gabius Apicius, who lived in the first century A.D. The three bolete recipes in this Roman cookbook can be translated as follows: "(1) Boil them, dry hot, and serve with wine sauce [*oenogarum*] and pepper pounded with liquor; (2) use pepper, sweet boiled wine [*caroenum*], vinegar, and oil; (3) boil in salt and serve with oil, wine, and pounded coriander seed." Sound interesting?

These recipes were very simple when compared to others found in the book, although Apicius was known in his day for meals that were considered extravagant even in that time of gustatorial excesses. Perhaps the recipes were kept simple to minimize the chances of an aristocratic cook making a fool of himself in front of his reclining visitors while he prepared mushrooms in the boletaria.

When you collect boletes to eat, young firm specimens are best. Most boletes are fleshy and provide a good amount of food. The entire cap and stalk of young boletes are good to eat. Even in older specimens the stalk often remains tender. Among the species of *Leccinum,* the stem become fibrous and hard in maturity and should be discarded. A general rule in deciding whether or not to include the stalk with the caps in cooking is: if the stalk is soft and tender, use it; if it's hard and fibrous, don't. In large, older specimens of boletes, the tubes should be removed if they are soft and spongy. If, for example, the tube layer of a king bolete doesn't feel firm when you press it in with a finger, you should peel off the layer. Soft, spongy tubes give a mushroom dish a slimy consistency when cooked. However, even if the tubes are removed from a mature bolete, a large part of the cap remains which cooks to a most delicious, firm, and succulent texture.

Boletes may also be preserved by canning, pickling, or freezing after the mushrooms have been sautéed.

20 King Bolete   EDIBLE, DELICIOUS
Boletus edulis
("clod" "edible")

COMMON NAMES

King bolete, cèpe, steinpilz, prawdziwy grzyb, borowik, porcino, and many others.

WHAT IT LOOKS LIKE

Cap: generally 3 to 6 inches across, sometimes up to 1 foot in diameter; convex, shaped like a hamburger bun; at times slippery when wet, brown to red-brown. *Flesh:* solid; white, sometimes reddish just under the cap; does not change color when bruised. *Pore surface:* white at first, changing to yellow with a tinge of green; depressed just around stalk. *Stem:* 4 to 7 inches tall; same width along entire length, club-shaped, or with bulblike base; fine white reticulation on entire stem or only near the top; stipe color is white to pale brown; flesh solid, white, no color change when cut or bruised. *Spores:* deep olive-brown.

KEY FEATURES

Hamburger-bun-shaped cap, white reticulation on thick stem, white to yellowish pore surface. Grows most commonly on ground under evergreens or mixed evergreen-deciduous woods. A similar species, the bitter bolete, has a bitter taste, pink pores, and dark brown reticulation.

WHERE FOUND

Found throughout the United States under conifers, especially pines or conifer-hardwoods. One variety (*Boletus edulis*—variety *clavipes*) is also found under birch and aspen. A closely related, also edible species, *Boletus variipes*, is found in thin oak woods in the summer.

WHEN

Late summer and fall.

21 **Bitter Bolete**   INEDIBLE, BITTER

Tylopilus felleus
("pillow cap" "bitter")

COMMON NAME

Bitter bolete.

WHAT IT LOOKS LIKE

Cap: 2 to 12 inches across; broadly convex; tan to crust brown; smoth, dry to the touch, but slippery when wet; surface cracks in dry weather. *Flesh:* white. *Pore Surface:* white at first, pale pink, then deeper pink; pores stain brown when bruised or handled; often depressed at stalk. *Stem:* 2 to 6 inches tall, may be enlarged at base; dark brown reticulation; brownish, paler toward apex. *Taste:* very bitter. *Spores:* pink.

KEY FEATURES

The bitter taste, the pinkish pores in maturity, and the dark-brown reticulation easily distinguish this mushroom from the king bolete.

WHERE FOUND

Usually found singly or scattered on the ground or on very rotten evergreen wood in central and eastern United States.

WHEN

Mostly in the summer. Also in early fall.

22 Granulated Bolete   EDIBLE, VERY GOOD
Suillus granulatus

("hog" "covered with granules")

COMMON NAMES

Granulated bolete, butterball, rusty bolete, sticky bun, pine tree boletus, slippery jack.

WHAT IT LOOKS LIKE

Cap: 2 to 6 inches across; convex; sticky; pale pinkish tan, sometimes has cinnamon-brown mottling caused by hardening of sticky gluten on surface. *Flesh:* white, becoming pale yellow in age. *Pore Surface:* white when young, turning pale yellow. *Stem:* 1½ to 3 inches tall; white, may be yellow near apex, lower half becomes brownish and upper part yellow in age; reddish brown to tan "paprika" dots on top part of stalk, dots look like splotches of brownish paint and do not rub off. *Spores:* pale yellow-brown.

KEY FEATURES

The pale brown, sticky cap, white to pale-yellow pores, whitish stem covered with dots, and growing location under white pine are key characteristics. Other species closely related to the granulated bolete are associated with other evergreens. *Suillus brevipes*, the short-stalked butterball, has a short stem with no dots and a darker cap. It is found under two- and three-needled pines such as pitch pine, red pine, jack pine, and ponderosa pine. *Suillus albidipes*, another similar species, has a cottony white skirt that hangs from the edge of the cap when the mushroom is young. It is found under lodgepole pine in the West and under white pine in the East. Both species are edible.

WHERE FOUND

Grows under pines, especially white pine. One of the main species in pine plantations. Often found in large numbers. In Michigan, the most commonly collected bolete in total number of pounds. Although granulated bolete commonly forms mycorrhizae with white pine, it is also found under other pines and less commonly under other evergreens. In the West it is common under lodgepole pine.

WHEN

Most common in fall, although in some regions begins fruiting in late summer.

23 Painted Bolete   EDIBLE, DELICIOUS

Suillus pictus
("hog" "painted")

COMMON NAMES

Painted bolete, eastern white pine bolete.

WHAT IT LOOKS LIKE

Cap: 1 to 5 inches across; conic when young, becoming convex to nearly flat in age; covered with thick red hairs; deep red at first, fading in age, revealing yellow-brown surface between the hairs; skirt or veil fragments along edge of cap. *Flesh:* yellow, changing very slowly to reddish when cut or bruised. *Pore Surface:* yellow; pores angular, radiate out from stem; pores are large enough so you can see inside walls; bruises reddish brown; tubes don't readily separate from cap, often extend down stipe. *Stem:* 1½ to 5 inches tall; slender, about ¼ to ½ inch thick; the same width along entire stem or enlarged slightly toward base; streaked with red hairs over the lower part of the stalk. In youth, cottony white veil hides pore surface and extends from cap edge to stipe; later separates, leaving grayish hairy zone on stipe, stipe yellow above this zone. *Spores:* olive brown.

KEY FEATURES

Red mushroom with yellow pores with red hairs on the cap and stalk. Found under white pine.

WHERE FOUND

Very common under white pine wherever these trees occur in the United States. A similar edible western species (*Suillus lakei,* variety *pseudopictus*) is found under Douglas fir trees.

WHEN

Late summer and fall.

24 Admirable Bolete
Boletus mirabilis
("clod" "wonderful")

EDIBLE, DELICIOUS

COMMON NAME

Admirable bolete.

WHAT IT LOOKS LIKE

Cap: 3 to 6 inches across; convex; woolly, maroon-brown. *Flesh:* firm; white to yellow, sometimes reddish when bruised. *Pore Surface:* bright sulphur-yellow, mustard-yellow in age. *Stem:* 3 to 6 inches tall; club-shaped to bulbous; up to 2 inches wide near base; dark brown; sometimes reticulated at apex; smooth to rough to shallowly pitted toward base. *Spores:* olive-brown.

KEY FEATURES

The maroon-brown cap and bright yellow pores coupled with the unusual occurrence of a bolete growing on wood are distinctive characteristics.

WHERE FOUND

Common on rotting coniferous logs or stumps or in the soil. Found mainly in the Pacific Northwest and Rocky Mountain states. Becomes rare farther east in the central states. Occurs on logs of fir, hemlock, and western red cedar, though most commonly on hemlocks.

WHEN

Fall.

25 Orange Bolete   EDIBLE, VERY GOOD

Leccinum aurantiacum
("of the oak" "orange")

COMMON NAMES

Orange bolete, brick cap, orange cap.

WHAT IT LOOKS LIKE

Cap: 2 to 8 inches across; convex like a hamburger bun; rusty red to reddish brown; surface feels like dry felt; cap covering (cuticle) hangs over edge of cap like extra material. *Flesh:* white, thick, firm; bruises slowly to gray with reddish overtones, then bluish gray. *Pore Surface:* tiny pinholes; at first white, becoming gray to dingy brown in age; bruises olive-red-brown; depressed around stipe. *Stem:* 4 to 8 inches tall; chunky; often narrowed at base and apex; white, covered with tufts, pale at first, becoming black or dark brown with age; flesh fibrous, white, becoming slowly gray with reddish to blue overtones. Flesh color change in mushroom most pronounced in the stem. *Spores:* brown.

KEY FEATURES
Large, rusty red cap with a robust white stem covered with sooty particles, a color change in the flesh, and occurrence under aspen and pines. Another orange- to red-capped mushroom (*Leccinum insigne*) fruits under aspen but in late spring and early summer. Once considered an earlier variety of *Leccinum aurantiacum*, this mushroom has now been made a separate species. Also very good to eat.

WHERE FOUND
Grows mostly under pines and aspen throughout the United States. Also found under other conifers, such as spruce and fir. After a good fall rain, this mushroom may form a huge carpet in aspen forests.

WHEN
Late summer to fall.

26 Red-pored Bolete   POISONOUS
Boletus subvelutipes
("clod" "almost velvet feet")

COMMON NAME
Red-pored bolete.

WHAT IT LOOKS LIKE
Cap: 2½ to 6 inches across; convex; yellow-brown to red-brown; turns blue to blue-black when bruised. *Flesh:* yellow, becoming whitish; turns blue at once when cut or bruised. *Pore Surface:* red,

changes to blue, then blue-black. *Stem:* 2 to 4½ inches tall; equal in width or slightly enlarged toward base; pale yellow mottled with almost velvety red markings; turns blue to blue-black when bruised, flesh does too. *Spores:* dark olive.

KEY FEATURES

The blue-staining and red pores are immediate warning flags to stay away from this bolete. Although this species can be confused with other blue-staining, red-pored boletes, it does not matter because all boletes that have either red pores, stain blue, or do both should be avoided. Several are known to be poisonous.

WHERE FOUND

Found singly or scattered under hardwoods or in mixed hardwood-evergreen woodlands in eastern North America south to Virginia.

WHEN

One of the first boletes to fruit, starting in early summer and continuing into fall.

Hen of the Woods

(*Polyporus frondosus*)

Many-capped Polypore

(*Polyporus umbellatus*)

When the hen of the woods first appears in the fall, newspapers often carry photographs of smiling mushroom collectors proudly displaying these desirable specimens (Figure 26). The large size of the smoky gray and white fungus known as the hen of the woods piques the curiosity of mushroomer and nonmushroomer alike.

Specimens of this fungus may grow up to 2 feet or more in diameter and weigh as much as 100 pounds. In his book *Mushrooms and Toadstools*, John Ramsbottom cites old records stating that "a specimen gathered near Leva, Hungary, was so large that it filled a two-horse cart." However, the typical hen of the woods (*Polyporus frondosus*) that you will find growing at the base of trees or stumps will generally be about a foot or so in diameter.

To the imaginative eye, a clump of the fungus looks like a setting hen that has just fluffed its feathers after being disturbed on the nest (Figure 27); thus, the mushroom's common name. The fluffed feathers are actually smoky gray to brown mushroom caps that grow at the tips of short white-stems (Figure 27 and Color Plate 27). The caps grow so close together that the short stems aren't visible to an observer standing over a mushroom clump. One must bend down to view the pure white underside of the mushroom and the small stems. The underside of the caps

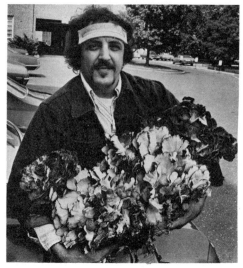

FIGURE 26. *Frank Petro of Watertown, Connecticut, holds a 40-pound hen of the woods. Petro also collected about 4 bushels of smaller hen of the woods, or cauliflower mushrooms as he calls them, on this same mushroom hunt.*

contrasts beautifully with the gray top. The white layer is dotted with holes or pores (hence, the Latin name *polypore*, "many pores"). Unlike its close relative, the sulphur shelf (*Polyporus sulphureus*), the hen of the woods has pores that can easily be seen without a hand lens.

The hen of the woods grows in the ground and at the base of trees, near but not on stumps and exposed roots. The fungus is a mild parasite of oak and other hardwood trees. The mycelium of the hen of the woods penetrates the roots and the base of a tree for several years, producing a white rot in the wood. The mycelium then spreads into the soil, forming masses that bind soil particles together. The fruiting hen of the woods springs up from these mycelial masses in the soil.

Once you find a hen of the woods, you can go back to the same spot to collect the mushroom year after year. I have a favorite spot, the base of a tall skeletal tree that was once a living oak. In late September, after heavy rains, I bicycle past the tree during my daily lunchtime checkup of foraging areas. Almost like clockwork, the mushroom can be seen coming up through the fallen leaf cover during the last week of September. Two large hen of the woods, growing about a foot apart, arise from the soil; one nearly hugs the base of the dead tree; the other grows near the flank of a large exposed root. After work, I return and collect the

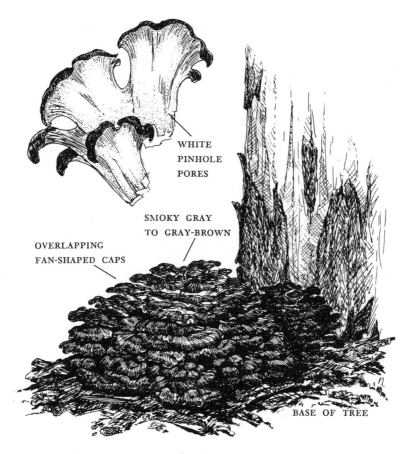

WHITE
PINHOLE
PORES

SMOKY GRAY
TO GRAY-BROWN

OVERLAPPING
FAN-SHAPED CAPS

BASE OF TREE

FIGURE 27. *Key features of the hen of the woods* (Polyporus frondosus)

mushroom, which becomes part of our evening meal.

Polyporus frondosus is a favorite fungus among Italian Americans. They call it the cauliflower mushroom because of its resemblance to the many-branched vegetable. This large fungus may be seen for sale in markets in Italian sections of cities, such as in Boston. On Federal Hill, in the Italian area of Providence, Rhode Island, the hen of the woods is also served in restaurants. The descendants of Italian immigrants carry on a tradition that goes back many years when this prized edible was sold in the markets of Rome. In Italy, this mushroom has been so highly prized that the mycelia of the hen of the woods were often allowed to grow unchecked in chestnut orchards. The fungus was held in more

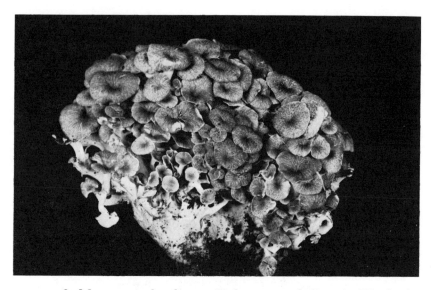

FIGURE 28. *Many-capped polypore* (Polyporus umbellatus). *The Latin name for the mushroom* umbellatus *means "umbrella."*

esteem than the chestnuts that grew on the host trees.

A rare mushroom that is similar to *Polyporus frondosus* is the many-capped polypore, *Polyporus umbellatus* (Figure 28). This mushroom also grows around stumps or old trees, is also edible, and is said to be equal in flavor to the delicious hen of the woods. The pale to smoky-brown caps of the mushroom are smaller than those of the hen of the woods and are round and depressed in the center; the cap of the hen of the woods is flat and fan-shaped. *Polyporus umbellatus* appears much earlier than the hen of the woods, fruiting in early summer throughout the northern United States and Canada. During most summers, this mushroom is very rare; however, it is more common during an unusually wet summer. Both mushrooms are equally excellent and edible.

A debate sometimes occurs between fans of the hen of the woods and devotees of another polypore, the sulphur shelf; each side claims its mushroom is better. Because of their similarity, the hen of the woods can be prepared in much the same way as the sulphur shelf mushroom. The hen of the woods is excellent sautéed in butter and served on toast, in casseroles, and as a substitute for chicken in recipes.

The entire clump of *Polyporus frondosus* can be eaten if it is tender throughout. If a knife passes through the mushroom as through butter, the mushroom is tender enough to eat. If you meet too much resistance in slicing through the entire mushroom, then use only the caps and stems that are tender. A typical hen of the woods provides more than enough mushrooms for one meal. What is left over can be preserved by pickling or freezing. To freeze the mushrooms, first parboil the entire mushroom in heavily salted water for ten minutes. Drain, slice into pieces, and pat dry. Insert pieces in freezer bags and place in the freezer. The hen of the woods is one of the few mushrooms that can be frozen without first sautéing, yet will retain much of its flavor when thawed.

27 Hen of the Woods   EDIBLE, DELICIOUS

Polyporus frondosus
("many pores" "leafy")

COMMON NAMES
Hen of the woods, cauliflower mushroom.

WHAT IT LOOKS LIKE
Fruiting Body: cluster of overlapping, fanlike caps; smoky gray to gray-brown, pure white pores underneath becoming yellowish in age; each cap ½ to 2½ inches across, caps arise from short white stems; forms a large cluster up to 2 feet in diameter. *Flesh:* white, pliable, looks like white chicken meat. *Spores:* white.

KEY FEATURES
Smoky gray overlapping caps with pure white underside forming a large cluster that grows in soil near the base of a tree or stump. A similar, rarer species (*Polyporus umbellatus*) has caps that are depressed in the center. The small stems are in the center of the cap and not off to the side as in the hen of the woods. Both species are edible and delicious.

WHERE FOUND

Usually grows singly, sometimes in twos or threes, in the ground at the base of a tree or stump. Although commonly found around oak, *Polyporus frondosus* also occurs near other hardwoods. Occurs generally in the United States east of the Great Plains.

WHEN

In fall after heavy rains.

Cauliflower Fungus

(*Sparassis radicata*)

Curly Sparassis

(*Sparassis crispa*)

What can weigh up to 50 pounds, looks like a bouquet of egg noodles, and is one of the safest mushrooms for beginners to identify? It's the cauliflower fungus (*Sparassis radicata*). The delicious mushroom is named for the cauliflowerlike branches that form a large, round clump at the base of evergreen trees. The flattened tips of the branches resemble lettuce leaves, egg noodles, or wavy ribbons, depending on who is looking at the fungus (Figure 29 and Color Plate 28). The tender "leaves" form large surface areas from which the spores of the fungus emerge. The spores are produced on both sides of the "leaves".

Although widely distributed, the cauliflower fungus is most common in the western part of the United States, particularly the Pacific Coast states and the Rocky Mountains. Virgin coniferous forest with stands of towering Douglas firs or other tall evergreens are a favorite habitat of the cauliflower fungus. When one of these edible fungi is discovered among large tree boles, there are likely to be exclamations of delight, for this creamy yellow to yellow-brown fungus is truly a prize find.

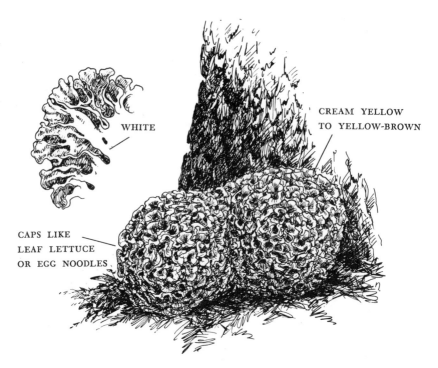

CREAM YELLOW
TO YELLOW-BROWN

WHITE

CAPS LIKE
LEAF LETTUCE
OR EGG NOODLES

FIGURE 29. *Key features of the cauliflower fungus* (Sparassis radicata).

The fungus generally ranges from the size of a softball to that of a basketball, although some specimens may reach a yard in width. The cauliflower fungus usually grows from 4 to 8 inches tall.

The mushroom is a parasite; it always grows at or near the base of an old living or dead evergreen tree because it parasitizes the tree's roots, causing a brown rot in the wood. The fruiting body itself arises and branches from a thick underground stalk that is attached to the conifer's roots. The stalk, or pseudosclorotium, is actually a thick mass of humus and soil particles bonded together by mycelia. The thick "umbilical cord" may thread its way more than 2 feet through the soil to reach a root. Sometimes the cauliflower fungus may be found growing on a log or stump. In such cases, no pseudosclorotium forms.

In the eastern part of the United States, a closely related species called the curly sparassis (*Sparassis crispa*) is found (Figure 30). This fungus, also delicious to eat, has thicker, larger leaves

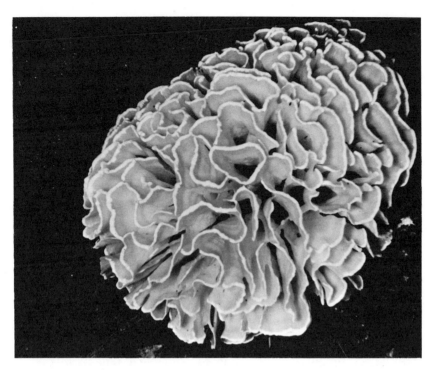

FIGURE 30. *Curly sparassis* (Sparassis crispa).

that rise nearly vertically from a common base and form wavy (curly) sheets that resemble ribbon candy. These wavy "leaves" or sheets (the mushroom's Latin name means "curly") have also been compared to the ruffled collars that appear in sixteenth- and seventeenth-century European and American portraits. The leaf surfaces have yellow-brown bands; the edges of the leaves are white. On the cauliflower fungus, no bands are present. The surface is uniformly colored cream-yellow to yellow-brown. The fungus, which is not common, grows at the base of pines and under oaks.

The cauliflower fungus is considered a choice find in many European countries. Although known as *Sparassis crispa*, it is not the same as our eastern curly sparassis. In fact, the European fungus is identical to the cauliflower fungus. In 1976, K. J. Martin and R. L. Gilbertson from the University of Arizona conducted a detailed study of cauliflower fungi (*Sparassis radicata*) from various western states; specimens of curly sparassis (*Sparassis crispa*) were also collected from the southeastern United States; and specimens of the so-called *Sparassis crispa* were obtained from European countries and from Japan. The botanists found that the European and Japanese *Sparassis crispa* specimens were the same as the cauliflower fungus (*Sparassis radicata*) of our western states. Eventually the *Sparassis radicata* of the American West may undergo a name change to *Sparassis crispa* to conform with the European mushroom, and another scientific name will have to be found for the eastern sparassis. Meanwhile, amateur mushroom hunters will continue to call the western species the cauliflower fungus, and the eastern species the curly sparassis. Both mushrooms will taste just as good no matter what their scientific label.

When collecting the cauliflower fungus, cut the fungus off at ground level. Don't pull it up, because you may also remove the deep, thick stalk (pseudosclorotium) attached to the tree root. To guarantee fruiting of this delicious edible from year to year in the same spot, the pseudosclorotium must remain intact. The cauliflower fungus will continue to fruit each fall as long as it obtains enough nutrients from the wood.

The cauliflower fungus can be kept fresh for a long time after it is picked. In Czechoslovakia, the base of young fruiting bodies is placed in water and stored in the cellar for several days. Sections are then cut from the mushroom as needed for a meal. Many meals can thus be obtained from one large fruiting body. Utilizing more modern conveniences, *Sparassis radicata* can be stored for weeks in an air-tight container in a refrigerator. Because of the large size of the mushroom, it is advisable to cut it into smaller pieces and store it in several containers.

Sparassis can also be preserved by drying, canning, or freezing. Before freezing, cut the sparassis into small pieces and sauté in butter or margarine. Charles McIlvaine in *One Thousand American Fungi* recommends drying a large sparassis intact and using it as a decorative object. Although it would certainly serve as a conversation piece, most mycophagists would prefer to eat the mushroom. Since the cauliflower fungus does not spoil readily or discolor in handling, some mycologists have recommended that it be cultivated commercially. In some European markets, cauliflower mushrooms collected from woodlands are sold. In San Francisco's Chinatown section, the mushroom is also seen for sale in the fall.

Sparassis is very good baked in a casserole or fried in batter. The fresh mushroom is strongly aromatic.

28 Cauliflower Fungus   EDIBLE, VERY GOOD
Sparassis radicata
("tear in pieces"   "rooted")

COMMON NAME
Cauliflower fungus.

WHAT IT LOOKS LIKE
Fruiting Body: large, round; resembles a rosette of egg noodles; generally 4 to 12 inches across; sometimes much larger; usually 4 to 8 inches high; many cauliflowerlike branches with lettucelike "leaves" at the tips arise from central stalk; cream-yellow to yellow-brown; odor pleasant. *Flesh:* white, firm. *Spores:* white.

KEY FEATURES
A large, round, lettucelike yellowish mass growing under evergreens, most commonly in the West.

WHERE FOUND
Grows under evergreen trees, on roots, never more than about 2 feet away from the tree's base. Attached to roots by a thick underground stalk. Sometimes may grow directly on log or on top of stump. Found in old-growth conifer forests in the western states. More common in the Pacific Northwest and Rocky Mountain states. Less common in central states and other areas.

WHEN
Fall.

Shaggy-Mane

(Coprinus comatus)

The shaggy-mane mushroom (*Coprinus comatus*), a large, very distinctive mushroom, has a cap that would arouse the envy of the shako-crowned honor guard at Buckingham Palace. The cap is barrel-shaped when young, is white to pewter in color, and has shaggy "hairs," which is why the mushroom is called shaggy-mane. The cap is perched on a slender stipe of purest white and grows to a stately 8 inches in height. A ring that can be moved up and down the stem also forms. The shaggy-mane does not maintain its shako shape during its entire existence. Later, the cap becomes bell-shaped, and eventually there is a third stage, which will be discussed later.

Although shaggy-manes may appear in the spring, they are primarily a fall mushroom. After a heavy rain, large clusters of these mushrooms may be seen on hard ground or in open, grassy areas such as lawns and golf courses. Ranks of these mushrooms numbering as many as a thousand may sometimes line roadsides and attract the attention of passing motorists. A host of shaggy-manes once crowded a midwestern baseball field, with one long line of the mushrooms cutting across the diamond from first base to left field.

The shaggy-mane is also a familiar sight in cities, springing up in vacant lots and parks, on hard-packed ground near side-walks, and on the small plots of land that city residents treasure as back yards or front lawns. The mushroom really lived up to its "city" reputation when naturalist Euell Gibbons, while teaching a course on wild foods, was challenged by his students to find enough wild edibles in New York City to make a meal. With the class in tow, Gibbons found a brushy area near 150th Street where hundreds of shaggy-manes grew. He diced the delicious mush-rooms, made a sauce for them, and then served up a pleasant repast to his admiring students.

The shaggy-mane has a reputation for tenaciousness and strength. It has been seen thrusting its narrow, egg-shaped head through blacktop, cracking or lifting a paving stone into the air, distracting tennis buffs by popping up through clay court surfaces, and growing in dumps full of cinder and other debris. In most of these cases, the shaggy-mane mycelium was present before an area was paved with blacktop or stone. When enough moisture seeped into the ground, fruiting bodies of the mycelium grew as usual and the relentless power of the expanding fruiting bodies was enough to lift a stone or to break through the hard macadam crust.

The distinctive, elegant look of the shaggy-mane makes it easy to identify. As mentioned earlier, it is one of the mushrooms designated by C. M. Christensen as the "foolproof four." My children and their friends instantly recognize the mushroom when it appears each fall even though it was pointed out to them only once.

A key characteristic in recognizing this mushroom has not yet been mentioned: the shaggy-mane cap turns to ink after it matures!

After the cap of the shaggy-mane passes from the barrel-shaped to the bell-shaped stage, the edges of the cap begin to turn black (see Figure 31, Color Plate 29). Then drops of ink appear. Gradually this remarkable transformation of the cap into ink continues upward until virtually the entire cap is gone. In the end, there has been a Dr.-Jekyll-and-Mr.-Hyde transformation, mycologically speaking. Only a few tattered remnants or the top-

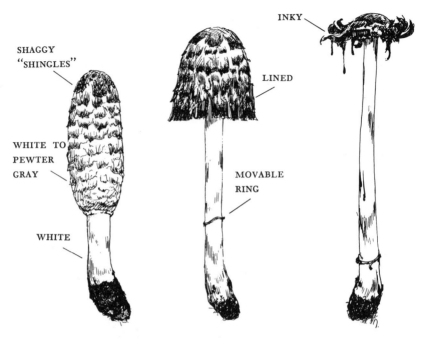

SHAGGY "SHINGLES"

WHITE TO PEWTER GRAY

WHITE

INKY

LINED

MOVABLE RING

FIGURE 31. *Key features of the drum major of the mushroom world, the shaggy-mane* (Coprinus comatus).

most part of the cap remains of what was once a stately mushroom. Percy Bysshe Shelley must have had the shaggy-mane in mind when he referred to a particular fungus in the garden of "The Sensitive Plant":

> Their mass rotted off them flake by flake,
> Till the thick stalk stuck like a murderer's stake,
> Where rags of loose flesh yet tremble on high,
> Infecting the winds that wander by.

Obviously Shelley was not a mycophagist and was not aware that this mushroom is considered one of the choicest edibles in the world of fungi (before it changes to ink, that is). Yet Shelley did correctly describe the mushroom as "infecting the winds that wander by." The cap change to ink helps ensure the dissemination of the spores into the air for future propagation of shaggy-manes. How? The gills of a shaggy-mane remain crowded close together like the pages of a thick book. The cap itself remains partly closed even during maturity, spreading out no more than a partially opened umbrella. Under these conditions, most maturing spores of the shaggy-mane simply would not have enough room to fall and be spread far and wide by the "infected winds" if it weren't for the inky process known as *autodigestion* or *deliquescence*.

Scientists have discovered that an enzyme triggers the process of self-destruction. The enzyme's action causes the cap to open slightly at the bottom edge. The gills also separate a bit. The spores in this region mature and fall just ahead of the advancing wave of blackening ink. As each part of the mushroom cap disappears in ink, another section of gills becomes exposed; more spores are liberated. Although many of the spores become engulfed by the advancing liquid ink, most of them escape into the air to "infect" the winds and eventually produce another crop of shaggy-manes for the mushroom collector.

The process of deliquescence is rapid. Various species of inky caps may mature in a few hours to a day. A mushroom collector must therefore collect shaggy-manes before they become inky. However, this is not a major problem, because in any clump of shaggy-manes, you will find the mushrooms in various degrees of maturity—from the youngest stage (when the mushroom looks like a cluster of elongated eggs) to the "tattered remnant" stage. You simply collect the ones that have not yet become inky.

Several species of mushrooms deliquesce; all are grouped under the genus *Coprinus* and are popularly called ink or inky caps. The French have a charming name for the inky caps; they call them *bouteilles à l'encre* which means "bottles of ink." Many of these species of inky caps grow in the United States. Two of the most common species, in addition to the shaggy-mane, are the glistening inky cap (*Coprinus micaceus*), a small, brown mushroom (Figure 32) that grows around stumps on buried wood in the spring and into fall, and the inky cap (*Coprinus atramentarius*), a chunky, gray species (Figure 33) that grows wherever organic material accumulates. Although both of these species are edible (as long as alcohol is not consumed with *Coprinus atramentarius*), they may be confused with other noninky, sometimes poisonous mushrooms. Therefore, beginners should limit them-

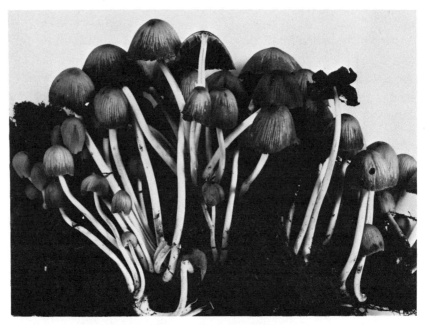

FIGURE 32. *Glistening inky cap* (Coprinus micaceus).

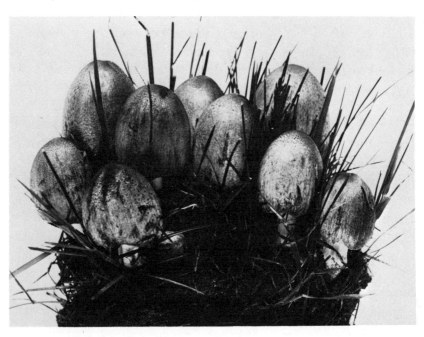

FIGURE. 33. *Inky cap mushrooms* (Coprinus atramentarius) *before the caps have turned to ink.*

selves among the inky caps to the "foolproof" shaggy-mane.

Once a delicious shaggy-mane or other inky cap has turned to ink, the mushroom's use to humans has not ended. In colonial days, ink was made from many plants, including inky cap mushrooms. In France, during the First World War, it was proposed that *Coprinus* ink be used as a substitute for the conventional ink, which was becoming more and more expensive. The potential usage of the ink of the inky cap mushroom has stimulated the imagination of many people. In his book *British Edible Fungi*, M. C. Cooke notes that "A curious proposal was made some years ago to utilize this ink for printing bank notes and other documents subject to forgery. The advantage being that at any period of time, by moistening the letters, the large spores would appear quite distinctly under the microscope, and the genuine ink at once determined. Ordinary ink, having no such origin, would present no such appearance."

Earlier, French botanist E. Boudier had come up with a novel way to present his research concerning the ink of the inky cap mushroom. In 1876, Baudier wrote the entire manuscript of his report with ink from the inky caps. Nearly all of the manuscript was written with *Coprinus atramentarius* ink. Only one paragraph was written with the ink from a shaggy-mane; that paragraph was devoted to a description of the shaggy-mane (*Coprinus comatus*). When the manuscript was exhibited at the Société Botanique de France, the president of the society thought that the ink was "très beau noir" (a very beautiful black) and impossible at first to distinguish from ordinary ink.

My curiosity was aroused after reading this, and I made some ink from shaggy-mane caps. I placed three large caps in a paper cup and let them sit overnight. Next day, a mini–Black Sea filled half the cup while three bumps—all that remained of the shaggy-manes—floated on top. The following day, even those top parts of the cap were gone. My children and I tried finger painting with the ink and writing sentences with a quill. Although the ink in the cup looked as if it had come from the blackest depths of outer space, the script was much grayer. Most of the dark color is due to the black spores suspended in the liquid. While writing, the mycophagist in me kept thinking how a short while ago, this ink originated from some of the most delicious wild mushrooms that you can taste.

The transformation of shaggy-manes and other inky caps into ink apparently has sinister connotations for nonmushroomers. Early one fall Saturday morning, well before most New Yorkers are stirring, Françoise Pascual, a member of the New York Mycological Society, was collecting shaggy-manes in a vacant lot when she was startled, not by an attacker, but by a voice behind her, warning, "Don't eat those! They're poisonous." Turning around quickly, Françoise saw an old woman who had been watching from her apartment window. Even though the woman probably knew nothing about mushrooms, she just *knew* that those mushrooms must be poisonous because of the way they turned black.

Reflecting on this and other incidents, I have wondered if the old saying that "a mushroom is poisonous if it turns silver black" may have originated as someone watched pewter or silvery colored shaggy-manes turn black. The possibility gains further credence when you realize that some inky cap species can cause unusual symptoms if the mushroom is eaten while drinking an alcoholic beverage. The temporary symptoms range from a rapid heartbeat and a flushed face and neck to a tingling sensation in the arms and legs (see p. 28). It would be relatively easy for the uninitiated to believe that all inky caps, and eventually all mushrooms, cause illness. From such observations, myths are made.

The gastronomical appreciation of shaggy-manes, as with many other edible mushrooms, is not a recent phenomenon. The Romans were fond of shaggy-manes, according to British nineteenth-century author W. Houghton. In a survey of the use of fungi in Greek and Roman literature, Houghton discovered that Pliny (A.D. 23–79) wrote about an edible "white fungi whose head stems are similar in form to the caps of the Flamens." The Flamens were priests during the time of the Roman Empire. These caps, which appear on Roman coins and on wall sculptures, look very similar to shaggy-mane caps. "I know of no other edible fungus which so much resembles the figures of these priestly caps," concluded Houghton in an 1885 article in the *Annals and Maga-*

zine of Natural History. Today, shaggy-manes are still collected and eaten in many parts of Italy.

The choice shaggy-mane can be prepared in many delectable ways. It is delicious in a cream sauce, excellent with eggs, and a fine garnish for meat such as veal. It can be pickled, and makes a superb soup, as described in the recipe section of this book. When sautéed, the white pieces of mushroom look like white meat and emit a heady aroma of wild mushrooms that is almost enough to make you forsake forever the relatively bland commercial mushroom *Agaricus bisporus*.

Many mushroom books stress the need for immediately cooking the shaggy-mane before it changes to ink. One book (perhaps facetiously) suggests taking a frying pan and butter on a collecting trip to cook the shaggy-manes over a fire before they liquefy. I once saw a woman snipping glistening inky caps (*Corprinus micacus*) from the base of a stump and dropping the caps into a frying pan resting on the ground. Other books advise that you eat the mushrooms as soon as you get home, or at least sauté them to deactivate the enzyme before placing the mushrooms in the refrigerator. Otherwise, the shaggy-manes may liquefy in four to six hours. From my experience, the deliquescence countdown is not always that critical. I have collected shaggy-manes in the morning, put them in the refrigerator, then cooked them at night without losing one shaggy-mane to deliquescence. Apparently, the rate of deliquescence is influenced by the amount of water in the mushroom. When I pick shaggy-manes during a dry period that follows a heavy rain, the mushrooms may stay free of ink for a day or more. Shaggy-manes, however, that were collected during heavy periods of rain did turn to ink more rapidly. In either case there was not a rush-into-the-woods-with-a-frying-pan type of emergency.

Leon G. Schemenauer, a regional biologist for the Michigan Department of Natural Resources, has come up with a new way to keep shaggy-manes fresh up to eight days. The mushrooms are submerged in a container of cold water, weighted down with a plate to keep the mushrooms underwater, and then refrigerated. Apparently, the enzyme that triggers deliquescence does not operate in water, or at least needs oxygen from the air to proceed.

Some mushrooms that managed to bob up above the water became dark; those kept underwater remained as white on the eighth day as on the first, and were just as good.

I have eaten shaggy-manes at stages ranging from the "egg" stage through to the bell-shaped cap before it started to deliquesce. At all stages the mushrooms are delicious, although some people prefer them at the youngest stages.

29 Shaggy-Mane   EDIBLE, DELICIOUS
Coprinus comatus
("dung" "hair")

COMMON NAMES
Shaggy-mane mushroom, shaggy-mane, horse-tail mushroom, lawyer's wig, shaggy beard, inky egg.

WHAT IT LOOKS LIKE
Cap: 2 to 4 inches long; like narrow egg at first, expanding to bell shape; white to pewter gray; covered with shaggy scales that look like ruffled feathers and may become brownish in age; edge of cap becomes lined in age; cap eventually forms tattered remnant or becomes rolled up after deliquescence. *Flesh:* white, soft. *Gills:* crowded; white, tinged with pink before becoming black with spores and melting with deliquescence. *Stem:* 3 to 8 inches tall; slender; purest white; may be slightly larger at base; hollow; has ring after cap becomes umbrella-shaped, ring can be moved up and down stipe, ring is sometimes washed off by rain. *Spores:* black.

KEY FEATURES
The white to gray, shaggy, barrel-shaped cap that turns to ink is very distinctive; white stipe with a movable ring are further identifying characteristics.

WHERE FOUND
Forms groups or ragged lines on lawns, fields, waste places, in sawdust, and along roadsides in cities, suburbs, and countryside.

Several to a few hundred or even on unusual occasions up to a thousand may be found growing in one area. Looks like eggs or partially opened umbrellas rising above the blades of grass. Widely distributed throughout the United States and one of the first mushrooms collected by beginners because they are often found on people's lawns.

WHEN

Primarily fall, although also occurs in spring. Appears late in the fall.

Oyster, Lilac, and Angel Wings
(Pleurotus)

OYSTER MUSHROOM (*Pleurotus ostreatus*)
LILAC-SPORED MUSHROOM (*Pleurotus sapidus*)
ANGEL WINGS (*Pleurotus porrigens*)

Oyster mushroom season is late fall, when days are brilliantly clear, a chilling bite is in the air, and the sweep of the landscape becomes more prominent after most of the trees have been nearly shorn of their leaves. Although oyster mushrooms also appear in other seasons, fall is the best time to view them because the boles and stumps on which they grow are no longer in competition with the leafy·canopy and bushes, and the mushrooms stand out on these bare trunks like a series of overlapping shelves (Figure 34).

The oyster mushroom (*Pleurotus ostreatus*) is an attractive fungus. It has white, gray, or tan caps 1 to 6 inches wide that are shaped like a fan or oyster shell. The underside of the cap has large white gills that look like knife blades (Figure 35). The fleshy cap is either attached directly to the wood from the side or has a short stem that tapers slightly downward from one side of the cap before it connects with the log, stump, or trunk. The gills also continue down the short stem, which, though not present in the mushroom illustrated, is sometimes covered with downy white hairs that look like the hairs of a stuffed toy animal. The stem is usually off center. Unlike many fungi that grow on wood, the oyster mushroom is soft and pliant, and not tough, hard, or leathery.

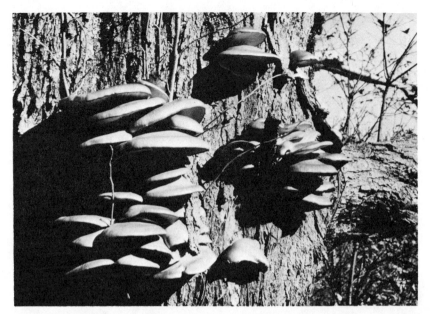

FIGURE 34. *Oyster mushrooms grow in clusters of fan-shaped caps like the lilac-spored mushrooms (above) shown on this sugar maple tree in the fall.*

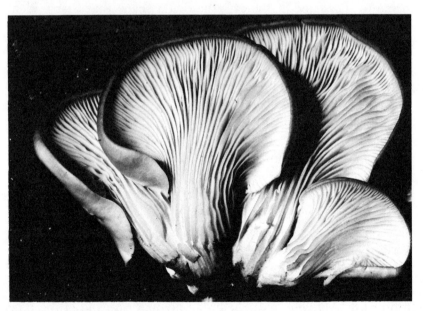

FIGURE 35. *The underside of an oyster mushroom. Note knife-edged white gills running down part of the short stem.*

The oyster mushroom can be found in woodlands as well as in any other areas where trees grow, including yards. It is found on both living and dead trees. On living trees, oyster mushrooms may be seen festooning a dead branch, growing out of a hole where a large branch may have been cut off, or forming a long line of overlapping, fan-shaped caps down a crease in the trunk of a dying tree. On the trunk of a dead tree or on a log or stump, clusters of oyster mushrooms are sometimes quite abundant. Each fall, I regularly visit a 50-foot-high bole of a dead tree that is covered nearly from tree top to root line with oyster mushrooms, clinging like barnacles to the hull of an old ship. Enough mushrooms are on this tree to supply many families with many meals. Trees laden with 40 to 50 pounds of oyster mushrooms or the similar lilac-spored mushroom (*Pleurotus sapidus*) are not that uncommon.

The oyster mushroom has sometimes been called the "shellfish of the forest." Several opinions exist as to how the oyster mushroom obtained its name. Although most books attribute the name to the shape of the cap, the oyster shape isn't that evident at first. From the top, the fan-shaped cap looks more like a clam shell. If you would attach an empty clam shell to a log at its hinge, it would look a lot like the oyster mushroom. To me, the oyster shape becomes evident only when a mushroom cap removed from a cluster is turned upside down. The stem of the cap, upside down, then looks like the small end of an oyster shell; the part where the cap spreads resembles the largest part of the oyster shell.

Some people think the oyster mushroom received its name because of its flavor; the taste, and even the slippery texture of the mushroom when eaten, mimics the oyster. A third reason may be the strong fragrance of the mushroom, a pleasant, strong odor. In an informal survey with the other four members of my family, I asked them to describe the odor of an object while their eyes were closed. With no idea that the odor test involved a clump of oyster mushrooms, all members described the smell as that of shellfish or fish. My wife said "shellfish"; my nine year old at the time said "dead clam"; my seven year old said "crab"; and the four year old said "fish." All the children were quite familiar with shellfish odors after summers spent shellfishing. When the survey was expanded to other people, most described the odor as "fishy," while other descriptions such as "sweet," "fruity," and "lemony" were also forthcoming.

Until recently, there has been some confusion in distinguishing between the oyster mushroom (*Pleurotus ostreatus*) and the closely related, and equally edible, lilac-spored mushroom (*Pleurotus sapidus*). In some books, both mushrooms are lumped together and called the oyster mushroom. This mushroom is described as having lilac-colored spores and as growing on a wide variety of trees, from maples to cottonwoods to aspen. The color of the cap is sometimes said to vary with the trees on which it grows. In other books, a distinction is made between *Pleurotus ostreatus* and *Pleurotus sapidus* according to the color of the spores. In the oyster mushroom, the spore deposit is described as white to creamy; in the lilac-spored *Pleurotus*, the spores are a pale lilac or lavender. This lilac color is so delicate that a spore print made from the cap of this mushroom looks like very faint, lilac-tinted brush strokes that radiate out in the shape of a fan. The strokes are actually made by the rows of spores where they fell from the gills. The heavier the spore fall, the more obvious the lilac tint. Sometimes the spore prints may at first seem white, but shortly after being exposed to the air, the color changes to lilac as the moisture in the spores evaporates.

To determine if the oyster mushroom and the lilac-spored mushroom were in fact different species, N. A. Anderson, S. S. Wang, and J. W. Schwandt of the University of Minnesota collected specimens from different trees in such widely separated states as New York, Minnesota, Ohio, and Louisiana. Aspen, oak, maple, hickory, elm, and basswood were the trees from which the mushrooms were collected. The scientists wanted to see if the spores of mushrooms from these trees would crossbreed. If the mycelia from the mushroom spores of one tree clamped together and merged with the mycelia from the mushrooms of another tree, then the mushrooms were considered one species. Such a merger is necessary for fruiting bodies to form.

The scientists found that the mushrooms fell into two groups. The mycelia from the various mushrooms collected from aspens crossbred readily; so did the mycelia of spores from the oak, maple, and other hardwoods. However, when mycelia of mushrooms taken from aspens were grown in the laboratory next to mycelia from the other hardwoods, they did not merge. In fact, a definite "zone of aversion" separated the two groups of mycelia.

The same grouping occurred when spore prints were taken of the mushrooms. The spore prints from the aspen turned out to be cream-colored; those from the other trees were all lilac-colored. The scientists concluded that the oyster mushroom (*Pleurotus ostreatus*) in this country is found only on aspen, while the lilac-spored mushroom (*Pleurotus sapidus*) grows on other hardwoods (Color Plate 30).

Because of the wide variety of trees on which *Pleurotus sapidus* grows, it is actually more common in many areas than the oyster mushroom. The mushroom that many people have been calling the oyster mushroom and collecting for many years turns out to be the lavender-spored *Pleurotus*. In fact, the University of Minnesota researchers note that if aspen had not been included in their study, they would have concluded that the oyster mushroom was either absent or rare in North America. Whatever the name, the mushrooms are still identical in appearance to a beginner, with the exception of spore color.

In their research, the scientists also discovered why the caps of these mushrooms differ in color. The more light that shines on the caps, the darker they become. "When we grew both species under low light intensities," the researchers note in the January–February, 1973, issue of *Mycologia*, "the pileus [cap] was white to cream color, but as the light intensity was increased, both species became gray to blue gray, and with increased light in a greenhouse there was some tint of light brown." I have seen a similar difference in *Pleurotus sapidus* growing in the fold of an old tree trunk. The mushrooms formed a garland down a crack in the fold. Where exposed to the sun, the *Pleurotus sapidus* was a light gray-brown; however, where some of these mushrooms were hidden from the sun by a large patch of bark, the caps were pale cream.

The lilac-spored and oyster mushrooms have a long growing season. They fruit repeatedly during the course of a year in wet weather, appearing commonly even in the spring, which is generally considered the morel season. However, fall is the best time to introduce a beginner to these mushrooms; not only are they more obvious during the leafless season, but they are also more abundant. In addition, the chances of finding beetles in between the gills are lessened during the colder weather.

When you search for oyster and lilac-spored mushrooms in the fall, you may find yourself in the woods with other sorts of hunters. In order to avoid the possibility of accidentally becoming someone's trophy, it is best to limit your search to those mushrooms on trees along back roads, or even in yards or posted woods. A drive along the byways will reveal a surprisingly large number of *Pleurotus sapidus* on trees near the road. Once you find particular sites where these mushrooms grow, record them in your notebook so that you can come back regularly to collect the mushrooms. Not only will these mushrooms fruit from year to year in the same place, but they will also fruit several times during the year after a rain.

The oyster and lilac-spored mushrooms can be considered mildly parasitic because they will invade a living tree that has been weakened by disease or by a storm. The aspen seems to be an ideal tree for the invading spores of *Pleurotus ostreatus*. It has soft, brittle wood that is easily damaged by wind, ice, and snow. It is a fast-growing, short-lived tree that is prey to many diseases. Aspen can almost be considered a "weed" tree, since they sprout up like weeds in wooded areas where trees have been cut down or swept by fire. It grows on sandy or rocky soils, often in prodigious numbers. In Colorado, the aspen are so numerous that the state seems awash in gold when the round green leaves turn golden in the fall. The aspens are a distinctive tree, with a pale greenish-white bark that looks like the bark of a birch tree, and leaves that stir easily in the slightest breeze. The popular name of the common aspen is the "quaking aspen."

Once an aspen has been damaged or weakened in some way, the invasion of the oyster mushroom may be extremely rapid. A severe winter storm once broke many branches in a forest of aspens, leaving open wounds on the trees. Spores from oyster mushrooms landed in many of these openings and the following year, a rich crop of *Pleurotus ostreatus* was seen growing out of these wounds. The white clumps of *Pleurotus ostreatus* are easy to spot in aspen woods, even from a moving car, in spring or fall. Once you are familiar with the oyster and lilac-spored mushrooms during the fall season, you can resume collecting the following spring.

Oyster mushrooms play a beneficial role in nature, helping to recycle a tree or stump back to the soil from whence the tree came. The oyster mushroom's persistence in decomposing wood must have achieved some kind of record when a cluster of these mushrooms was found in 1977 growing out of an old kitchen chair that had been stored for some time in a dark basement of a Grass Valley, California, home. "Both the plastic and the padding had cracked in one corner," said resident Lillian Mott, "allowing the *Pleurotus ostreatus* or oyster mushrooms to pop up from the wood base beneath where the spores must have dropped—no one knows how long ago." She added: "This must have happened before the tree went to the sawmill and survived the process of making it into lumber."

The oyster and lilac-spored mushrooms are extremely hardy, surviving in severe weather that would affect less hardy organisms. I have seen delicate ice crystals on the gills of *Pleurotus sapidus* on a cold fall day while hoarfrost or ice crystals bearded or glazed the top of the caps. Nature seems to provide its own deep-freeze preservation of these mushrooms until a collector comes along. These fan-shaped mushrooms may even appear during a thaw in the coldest winter months in the northern part of the country.

A winter bloom of oyster mushrooms once saved the day for an annual dinner of the New York Mycological Society when John Cage, composer and founding member of the society, spotted a frozen clump of lilac-spored mushrooms and collected them. The year had been a lean one for society collectors, who usually preserve wild mushrooms and serve them in various ways at the annual dinner and tasting. As it turned out, the mushrooms brought in by Cage were the only wild mushrooms prepared at the dinner. To collect the mushrooms, which were frozen solid to a tree, Cage related now he diligently attacked the clump from high on a ladder "with all sorts of weapons including an ice pick and a saw." But he couldn't budge the mushrooms. Cage then borrowed an ax from some construction workers on a nearby project, then clambered up the ladder, and chopped off some of the mushrooms. He collected enough to provide sixty dinner members with a steaming bowl full of rich, meaty, succulent "funghi bordelaise," which turned out to be the gastronomic highlight of the evening. When the ax was returned to the construction workers, Cage offered them some of the frozen mushrooms, but they quickly demurred.

Can the oyster or lilac-spored mushroom be confused with any other fungi that grow on wood? Yes. One species is the bear mushroom (*Lentinellus ursinus*). Like the *Pleurotus ostreatus* and *sapidus*, this mushroom (Figure 36) has a fan-shaped cap, is gilled, and grows on wood, including logs and stumps of hardwoods and evergreens. When young, the cap is whitish and could possibly be confused with the two pleurotus species. However, the similarity ends with these characteristics. The bear mushroom also has several other key characteristics that should easily differentiate it from the oyster and lilac-spored mushroom. First, the edge of the gills, which are pinkish, are ragged like the teeth of a saw, while the *Pleurotus ostreatus* and *sapidus* have white gills that are as smooth as a knife edge. The top part of the cap is also hairy where it attaches to a stump or log; when mature, the hairs form a distinctive dense brown mat that looks just like the fur of a brown bear. And finally, a simple test (a nibble, not a swallow) will quickly help you distinguish between this mushroom and the other two species. Although the bear mushroom is not poisonous, it has an extremely bitter taste. When I found this mushroom for the first time on a foray, the field-trip leader asked all of us to sample the mushroom. The bitter taste that burned the tongue almost numb was a telling way to remember this species forever. For some people, it takes a few seconds before the bitter taste is noted. Although there are other species of *Lentinellus* found on wood, their serrated or saw-toothed edges always give them away.

Another *Pleurotus* species that may be confused with *Pleuro-*

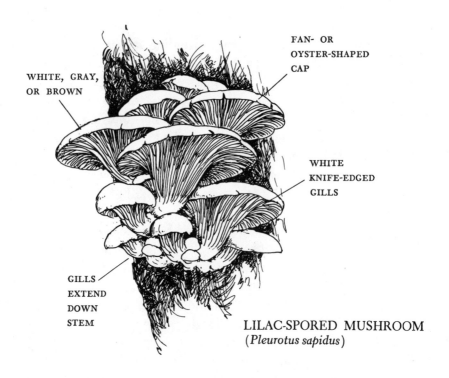

WHITE, GRAY, OR BROWN

FAN- OR OYSTER-SHAPED CAP

WHITE KNIFE-EDGED GILLS

GILLS EXTEND DOWN STEM

LILAC-SPORED MUSHROOM
(*Pleurotus sapidus*)

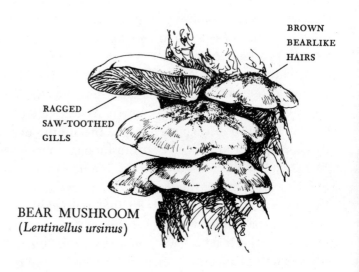

BROWN BEARLIKE HAIRS

RAGGED SAW-TOOTHED GILLS

BEAR MUSHROOM
(*Lentinellus ursinus*)

FIGURE 36. *Key features of a lilac-spored mushroom* (Pleurotus sapidus) *and a look-alike, the bear mushroom* (Lentinellus ursinus).

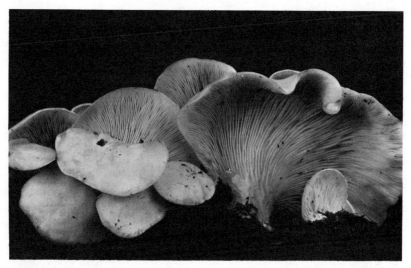

FIGURE 37. *Angel wings* (Pleurotus porrigens).

tus ostreatus and *sapidus* is the small, beautiful, and fragile angel wings (*Pleurotus porrigens*). This pure white mushroom (Figure 37) grows on old, mossy evergreen logs, especially hemlock, in the northern United States and along the Pacific coast. When seen against the lush, green moss and lichens mantling an ancient hemlock log, these snow-white mushrooms with the frequently lobed or wavy (when mature) caps can be said to resemble angel wings. The angel wings are much smaller (1 to 3 inches wide) than the other two *Pleurotus* mushrooms. The flesh is also very thin and pliant, and the gills are more crowded in the angel wings. The mushroom also does not have a strong odor as the other mushrooms do. The spores of the angel wings are white. Because it is edible, you don't have to worry about confusing this species with *Pleurotus ostreatus* and *sapidus*. In fact, some people think angel wings is better tasting than the other two mushrooms. Others use the mushrooms as a filler to provide bulk to a mushroom meal when pickings have been lean. Because angel wings grow in such large numbers, it doesn't take long to accumulate many of these small mushrooms.

To make doubly sure that you have a *Pleurotus*, whether it be the oyster mushroom, the lilac-spored mushroom or the angel wing, take a spore print the first few times you collect these fungi.

If the spores are white, cream, or lilac-tinged, and they look like the drawings or photos in this book, then you have a *Pleurotus*. It is important for you to remember that no known *Pleurotus* species with such spore colors are poisonous. The spore print will rule out other groups of mushrooms with stemless or off-center stems that grow on wood (for example, *Crepidotus* has brown spores, and *Gymnopilus* has yellowish-brown spores). Taking the spore print when you are in the field is easy to do and need not interrupt your collecting for more than a few seconds. Simply put a mushroom cap face down on a piece of paper in a waxed sandwich bag (See Part I, "In Pursuit of Mushrooms.") and place the bag in the bottom of your basket. Put the remaining tentatively identified "*Pleurotus*" mushrooms in a separate bag for possible later use in the pot. By the time you finish mushrooming and collecting shaggy-manes, boletes, or other fall provender, the spore print should be ready for you to inspect. If you have a white, cream, or lilac spore print, and the mushroom matches the photos and drawings in this book, then you will have safely ruled out other wood-inhabiting species that may be inedible.

The oyster mushroom is increasingly being cultivated in the home as well as commercially. Fresh cultivated oyster mushrooms are available in stores on the West Coast and in other regions where amateurs are selling the mushrooms grown in their homes or garages. A typical example is Louis Agro of Hamilton, Ontario. Agro has been growing *Pleurotus ostreatus* on bales containing a mixture of straw, paper, cornmeal, and haymeal. Before this mixture is formed into bales, it is first pasteurized and oyster mushroom spawn is then added. The bales are then stacked in vertical rows like tree trunks against the wall of a converted garage. A crop of oyster mushrooms appears every twelve to fourteen days, and the mushrooms continue to fruit periodically for five to eleven months. Agro has no trouble selling all the mushrooms he produces at the Hamilton market.

In addition to Canada and the United States, the oyster mushroom is also cultivated in Europe, Taiwan, and Australia. It can also be grown in the home from mushroom kits containing a small log impregnated with spawn. In Germany, some collectors haul stumps containing oyster mushrooms onto their land and periodically water the wood to obtain repeated fruitings.

The oyster and lilac-spored mushrooms can be prepared in several ways. Many people feel they are best suited to casserole-type dishes that require long, slow cooking. The North American Indians probably used these mushrooms to make a kind of porridge. In a visit to Indian tribes in the eighteenth century, a Jesuit named Rale described in a letter to his brother how white tree fungi were "cooked and reduced to a sort of porridge." However, the taste of the mushroom must have been quite foreign to Jesuit Rale's taste because he claimed that the dish was "very far from having the flavor of porridge."

In an article on the "Use of Plants by the Indians of the Missouri River Region," published in the 1911–1912 report of the Bureau of American Ethnology, Melvin Randolph Gilmore tells how the Indians of the Dakota nation relished another white *Pleurotus (Pleurotus ulmarius)*, a relative of the oyster mushroom. This fall mushroom, which has a scaly cap and a cottony stem, frequently grows high in a tree out of knotholes and branch stubs. Gilmore relates seeing Indian women "gathering it in a grove of boxelder near the place where the Cannonball River flows into the Missouri River. . . . They were looking for it in decayed spots caused by tapping the trees for the purpose of sugar making, for these people still make sugar from the sap of the boxelder." When young and tender, notes Gilmore, the mushroom is most delicious.

When you are gathering the oyster and lilac-spored mushrooms to eat, collect young and tender caps. Cut away the stem if present because it can be tough. Make sure no beetles are present in the folds of the gills. If they are, soak the mushrooms in cold, salted water; the beetles will desert the mushrooms and float to the top. The mushrooms can then be dabbed dry.

The association of the oyster mushroom with shellfish has inspired some chefs to prepare the mushrooms as one would prepare seafood dishes. Margaret Lewis of the Boston Mycological Club has substituted these mushrooms for oysters in many dishes and has fooled many food experts. The tender parts of oyster mushrooms may also be dipped in an egg batter, rolled in bread or cracker crumbs, and fried. The mushrooms taste like fried oysters and when prepared this way, says Charles McIlvaine; "they are not excelled by any vegetable and are worthy of a place in the daintiest menu." California mycologist Robert T. Orr even has a cat who is fond of fried oyster mushrooms but will ignore other mushrooms. Apparently the cat with a fondness for fish or shellfish was fooled by this mushroom in shellfish disguise.

The oyster mushroom has been used in various Oriental dishes and in stews, soups, and casseroles. The oyster and lilac-spored mushroom can be preserved best by canning and freezing after sautéing.

30 Lilac-spored Mushroom   EDIBLE, VERY GOOD
Pleurotus sapidus
("side ear"   "savory")

COMMON NAMES
Sapid mushroom, lavender-spored pleurotus, oyster mushroom, willow pleurotus, lilac-spored mushroom, lilac-spored pleurotus.

WHAT IT LOOKS LIKE
Cap: 1 to 6 inches across; shaped like fan, oyster, or even modern helmet-shaped street lamp; smooth; convex; color varies from white, gray, tan, to darker brown. *Flesh:* white. *Gills:* white, knife-edged, fairly well separated, forked, extend down stem. *Stem:* short, if present; white, stout, firm, solid; sometimes covered with downy white hairs like those of stuffed toy animal; attached to side of cap, and tapers downward from cap; may be off center. Odor of shellfish. *Spores:* lilac.

KEY FEATURES
Fan- to shell-shaped caps that usually form overlapping shelves; white, knife-edged gills that extend down stem; lilac spores. Grows on various hardwoods. The oyster mushroom (*Pleurotus ostreatus*)

is identical except that it has creamy spores and grows only on aspen.

WHERE FOUND

On stumps, logs, and trunks of dead hardwoods and living trees that have been weakened by disease or storm damage. Both the oyster mushroom and the lilac-spored mushroom are widely distributed and common.

WHEN

Spring, in the summer after heavy rains, fall, and even in winter during thaws.

Winter

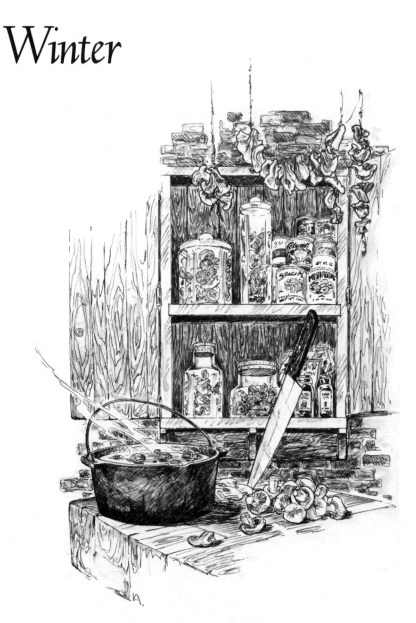

Winter is the quiet season for mushroomers in most parts of the country. Though the mushroom collecting season still lingers on the West Coast and in other warmer areas, collecting in the colder regions is limited to the oyster or lilac-spored mushroom or the velvet-stemmed or winter mushroom (*Flammulina velutipes*) that sprout from trees during winter thaws. However, the farsighted mushroomer will have preserved some of the mycological fruits collected during the peak seasons. Morels that were dried in the spring are excellent when reconstituted with milk or water. The freezer should be crammed with sautéed mushrooms such as the meadow mushroom or chunks of hen of the woods or sulphur shelf mushrooms. Perhaps jars of pickled shaggy-manes sit on the shelf within easy reach to be used an appetizer. Whatever the preservation method, now is the time to enjoy these mushrooms during this respite from collecting. Of course, you're not limited to the wild mushrooms that you have preserved. You can also purchase mushrooms from Oriental stores or specialty shops, or you can grow mushrooms from do-it-yourself kits (see Part III for more information on these two subjects). While I look out the kitchen window, framed by frost crystals, I think of my fellow mushroomers on the West Coast clambering over the snow-free slopes of California, looking for edible mushrooms. As an old Red Sox fan stuck in snow-swept New England, I can only murmur "Wait till next year. . . . "

Part III

Mushrooms for the Table

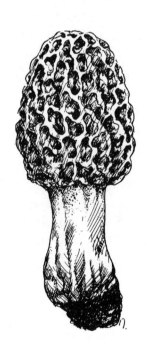

For a mycophagist, the supreme moment (after finding a favorite mushroom) comes when with fork in hand and a mushroom nugget deliciously cooked, the finder sends it on its way to the mouth. To those who have eaten the nutty cèpe or the woodsy morel, it is truly a moment to be savored. However, before this delightful part of the mushroom's journey from woods to mouth is completed, there are many paths in mushroom cookery that can be taken. One may be short—the simple sautéing of the mushroom in olive oil or butter—or the path may be more divergent, with mushrooms immersed in a bubbling casserole or spread in a rich cream sauce over meat or fish. One method of preparation not to be recommended, however, was supposedly favored by Russian Cossacks to make some of the tougher species of wild mushrooms more tender. The fierce-riding Cossacks, so the story goes, inserted tough mushroom caps between the saddle and the flank of the horses on which they rode. After a day of rough riding, the battered mushroom caps would certainly be tender, although I don't think that I would try the mushrooms despite my adventuresome palate. Whether the story should be taken with several grains of salt does not matter. What it does illustrate is that wild mushrooms may be prepared in many ways.

In this part of the book, various methods of preparing and preserving wild mushrooms are described to introduce you to the delicious and wide-ranging tastes of wild mushrooms. Your repertoire of exotic mushrooms will also be greatly expanded with the Part III section "Stalking Wild (and Not So Wild) Mushrooms in Stores." You will learn how more than a dozen kinds of mushrooms from different parts of the world can be purchased in stores or by mail. And, finally, the section "Growing Your Own Mushrooms" will show you how you can easily cultivate many wild species on your lawn, in your woodland, and even in your home.

Recipes
for All Seasons

Here are some helpful hints to review before preparing any species of mushrooms. As described earlier, the mushrooms that you have brought home in your basket should already be quite clean. When the mushrooms were picked, the base of any stipe containing soil should have been cut off and any leaves, needles, or other debris should have been wiped off the cap. Mushrooms that are old, water-logged, insect-infested, or partly decayed should also have been left behind in the woods. Only the youngest, firmest, and freshest mushrooms should be in your basket.

If the mushrooms still need to be cleaned, use a damp cloth, brush, or absorbent towel to wipe them off. Avoid washing mushrooms, if possible, because washing causes them to lose some of their flavor and makes them soggy. If mushrooms must be washed, do it quickly in cold water. Dry the mushrooms immediately with a paper towel.

The caps of mushrooms should not be peeled, unless the cap cuticle is sticky (as in the granulated bolete) or too deeply imbedded with dirt. Much of the flavor is in the cuticle. Stipes should be cut off if they are tough or stringy. Some stipes, such as the chunky stem of the king bolete, are very good to eat. These may be cut up and sautéed with the caps or cooked separately and used in soups or gravies.

Generally, mushrooms should be cooked quickly over low heat. Too much heat or cooking mushrooms for a long period of time will make them tough. However, firm or tougher types of mushrooms such as the chanterelle or the hedgehog mushrooms require longer and slower cooking.

The best way to learn how a particular mushroom tastes is to sauté the caps in a small amount of butter or margarine, gill side up first, to let the moisture evaporate. Then turn the caps over and sauté the other side. Mushrooms shrink a good deal in cooking. They should be salted only when they are almost ready. Unmasked by other seasonings, the essence of a mushroom comes through by simple sautéing.

An appealing way of obtaining the basic taste of a mushroom has been proposed by Charles McIlvaine, who suggests that you take a small vial of olive oil or a small container of butter and a mixture of salt and pepper along with you on your collecting expedition. When you find an edible mushroom, collect a few dry pieces of wood and start a fire. Then split a green stick at one end (he suggests using sassafras, birch, or spicewood), insert the mushroom in the cleft, and hold it over the fire. After adding the oil or butter and the seasonings, eat the mushroom. In America's distant past, the Indians may have indulged in such mushroom feasts, but instead of butter or olive oil, the added ingredients may have been bear fat or other oils from wild game.

Of course, the preparation of mushrooms need not be so puristic. Some mushrooms do have a delicate flavor that is easily overpowered by heavy seasoning. When cooking these mushrooms, the mushroom flavor should predominate. However, other mushrooms (such as puffballs) do benefit greatly by the addition of a variety of flavors. And some mushrooms have such a dominant flavor that even the addition of many ingredients will not ruin the mushroom dish.

Preparing mushrooms is much like playing a symphonic theme with its many variations. The main theme in wild-mushroom cookery might be to sauté the mushrooms in butter, oil, or margarine with perhaps a dash of lemon juice. The variations, in the case of the cèpe, for example, would be to add shallots to mushrooms sautéed in oil (cèpes bordelaise) or to add garlic to cèpes in butter (cèpes provençal). For other mushrooms, the variations might include sour cream, parsley, or Parmesan cheese. Whatever preparation is chosen for a particular species, the result is a variety of tastes for the mycophagist with an emphasis on the mushroom.

Recipes for the species or groups of mushrooms described in detail in Part II of this book are given here in seasonal order. The recipes, a sampling and not an encyclopedic collection, were specifically chosen to bring out the best in these particular mushrooms. In several cases a different species may be substituted, for each will contribute its own taste or texture to the recipe. The recipes were obtained from many sources, ranging from mushroom cookbooks published by local mycological societies to recipes handed down through generations in one family. In several cases, recipes have been improved by the sure eye of my wife who can often immediately realize a recipe's potential (or fault) by simply reading the list of ingredients, while I her husband, who, may prepare many a mushroom recipe, would rather pass judgment on a dish by tasting it instead of preparing it. I'm more comfortable in the role of art critic than artist in matters of culinary expertise.

Spring

MORELS The splendid flavor of the highly prized morel should not be smothered with heavy flavorings or sauces. A morel may be simply sautéed in butter or its hollow interior can be stuffed with various fillings. It can be used in a cream sauce for beef or fish. Because of the many nooks and crannies in a morel's cap, which are ideal hiding places for sand, this mushroom should be washed quickly in cold water to remove the grit. The entire mushroom can be used. To stuff the mushroom, slice it in half; both hollow halves can then be stuffed. A recipe for stuffed morels and one for morels in cream sauce appear below. The stuffed-morel recipe is from the New Jersey Mycological Association's *Mycophagist's Corner*, a booklet of recipes.

MORELS IN CREAM SAUCE

¼ lb. butter	salt and pepper to taste
1 lb. morels, sliced	¼ cup flour, sifted
pinch of salt	2 cups heavy cream
juice ¼ lemon	

Melt half of the butter in saucepan. Add morels with the lemon juice, a pinch of salt, and one twist of the pepper mill. Bring to a boil, tossing the mushrooms often. Cover and cook for 10 minutes. Drain morels, reserving the liquid. Melt the remaining butter in a saucepan and mix in sifted flour to make a smooth paste. Cook 3 minutes over low heat so that the flour doesn't burn. Remove from the heat and cool to room temperature. When cool, add the cream, stirring constantly with whisk, until the mixture thickens. Add enough of the reserved liquid to achieve the desired consistency. Correct seasoning. Add morels. Serve on toast or over rice. *Serves 4.*

STUFFED MORELS

4 large morels	½ cup puréed spinach
olive oil	3 tbs. butter, melted
1 small onion, minced	salt and pepper
½ cup minced ham	grated cheese

Slice the morels in half lengthwise, wipe the insides, dip the exteriors in oil, and place on a baking sheet. Mix the onions, ham, and spinach with the butter. Season to taste. Stuff hollows of the mushrooms with the mixture and sprinkle with cheese. Bake at 375° for 20 minutes. *Serves 4.*

Summer

CHANTERELLES AND HORN OF PLENTY The texture and flavor of the meaty chanterelle mushrooms are best brought out by long cooking at very low temperatures. Chanterelles are excellent in sauces, stewed with meat, or served on toast. The chanterelles-on-toast recipe appears in *The Wild Gourmet* by Babette Brackett and Maryann Lash. The fragrant, much thinner horn of plenty is delicious simply prepared with eggs.

CHANTERELLES ON TOAST

1 *cup chanterelles*	2–3 *tbs. dry white wine*
2 *tbs. butter*	¼ *cup beef bouillon*
1 *tbs. flour*	4 *slices toasted French*
¼ *tsp. salt*	*bread*
4 *grinds pepper*	

Clean and slice the chanterelles. Melt the butter over low heat. Stir in the chanterelles, and cook for 20 minutes, stirring every 5 minutes. Add the flour, and stir over medium heat for 2 minutes. Add the salt, pepper, wine, and bouillon, and stir until thickened. Serve over the French bread. This can also be used as a sauce over fish or chicken. *Serves 4.*

HORN OF PLENTY WITH EGGS

1 *tbs. chopped chives or*	2 *tbs. butter*
parsley	3–4 *large eggs*
½ *cup chanterelles or*	*salt and pepper to taste*
horn of plenty	

Chop the chives or parsley. Clean and slice the mushrooms. Melt butter in skillet, break eggs in bowl and whisk slightly. Add eggs to hot butter, stir quickly, then add mushrooms, herbs, salt, and pepper. Slide eggs onto a plate while they are still moist. *Serves 2.*

SULPHUR SHELF MUSHROOMS   Because of its chicken-like texture, this mushroom can be used in any recipe that would normally call for chicken. It is especially delicious in casseroles. The recipe below by Margaret Morris of Great Neck, New York, is the dish described earlier in the book in which a garden club member thought that she was eating chicken.

SULPHUR SHELF SNACK

1 *tbs. chopped onion*	1 *clove garlic, finely*
2 *tbs. butter*	*chopped*
2 *cups cleaned sulphur*	¼ *cup sour cream*
shelf mushroom pieces	1 *tsp. salt*
¾ *cup chicken broth*	2 *tbs. chopped parsley*

Sauté the onion in butter for 1 minute, add the mushrooms, and stir until the butter is absorbed. Add the broth, and cook 15 minutes or until the mushrooms are tender. Add the garlic, sour cream, and salt. Stir until well blended over low heat. Sprinkle with parsley, and serve with small toast rounds or crackers. *Serves 6 to 8 as a snack.*

MEADOW MUSHROOMS   The tasty meadow mushroom, which has a much stronger flavor than the commercial *Agaricus bisporus*, can be used as a substitute for any recipe in cookbooks calling for the cultivated mushroom. However, the recipe given here illustrates how good the meadow mushroom is raw in salads.

SPINACH-MUSHROOM SALAD

¾ *lb. fresh raw spinach*	*croutons*
½ *lb. meadow mushrooms*	*Poppy Seed Dressing*
2 *hard-boiled eggs, chopped*	
red onion rings	

Clean and dry spinach leaves. Tear them into bite-size pieces. Clean the mushrooms and slice thinly. Add to the spinach. Add eggs as garnish with onion rings and croutons. Add Poppy Seed Dressing and toss. *Serves 6.*

Poppy Seed Dressing:

¾ *cup sugar*   1½ *tbs. finely minced onion*
1 *tsp. dry mustard*   1 *cup salad oil*
1 *tsp. salt*   1½ *tbs. poppy seeds*
½ *cup cider vinegar*

Put the sugar, mustard, salt, and vinegar in a blender and combine. Add the onion, oil, and poppy seeds. Blend again. *Makes about 1½ cups.*

TEETH FUNGI The thick, firm hedgehog mushroom has a texture similar to that of a chanterelle so that it may be substituted in chanterelle recipes. It should be cooked slowly like the chanterelle. The white *Hericium* species, such as bear's head and the satyr's beard, have a mild taste and are usually served with vegetables. The Puget Sound Mycological Society recommends the following recipe:

BAKED MUSHROOMS WITH TOMATOES AND ONIONS

4 *tbs. butter*   *salt, pepper, Ac'cent to taste*
4 *cups sliced hedgehog*   2½ *cups chopped tomatoes*
  mushrooms   1 *cup fresh bread cubes*
1 *tbs. lemon juice*   *salt and pepper to taste*
2 *tbs. butter*   1 *cup buttered bread*
2 *medium-sized onions,*   *crumbs*
  sliced

Melt the butter in a skillet. Add the mushrooms. Sauté over medium heat for 5 minutes or until the liquid evaporates. Add the lemon juice. Remove from the skillet and reserve. In the same skillet, melt the butter. Add the onions, and sauté them until they are transparent. Place the onions in a baking dish. Cover with the sautéed mushrooms. Sprinkle with salt, pepper, and Ac'cent. Cook the tomatoes with the bread cubes. Add salt and pepper. Pour over mushrooms. Sprinkle buttered crumbs on top. Bake at 350° for 30 minutes. *Serves 6 to 8.*

PUFFBALLS These large mushrooms have a very subtle flavor that benefits from seasonings and herbs. Perhaps the most common way to prepare puffballs is to bread them. Some people add various seasonings to the crumbs. My favorite recipe, the second one given, is puffballs in sour cream with chives.

BREADED PUFFBALLS

1–2 *large puffballs*	*cracker crumbs*
2 *eggs*	*butter*
salt and pepper to taste	

Slice the puffballs about ¼ inch thick. Beat the eggs slightly and add salt and pepper. Dip both sides of puffball slices in egg mixture, then into cracker crumbs and sauté in butter until golden brown. *Serves 4 to 6.*

PUFFBALL WITH SOUR CREAM

1 *large puffball*	*salt*
chopped chives	*butter*
sour cream	

Slice the puffball thinly and sauté the slices in a small amount of butter. Stack the slices, putting between each layer a sprinkling of chopped chives and a layer of sour cream. Continue making the layers until the pile is about 5 inches high. Then cut it in half and serve. *Serves 4.*

Fall

BOLETES The sweet, nutty taste of the king bolete is so unique that is needs only to be sautéed in butter. However, *Boletus edulis* and the other boletes mentioned earlier can also be prepared in many other ways and still impart a delicious flavor to the dish. As an indicator of the universal appeal of the king bolete, three recipes from different countries are given here. One is French, one is Polish, and one is German.

CÈPES PROVENÇALS

1 lb. firm, fresh boletes	salt and pepper to taste
2 tbs. butter	2 tbs. fresh parsley, chopped
6 tbs. butter	French or Italian bread, sliced
2 cloves garlic, chopped	

Clean and slice the mushrooms. Then cook them in 2 tablespoons of butter, uncovered, until the mushrooms just begin to wilt (for 2 or 3 minutes). Remove the mushrooms from the pan and drain them. Add the drained, soft mushrooms to the remaining butter, which has been melted and is hot, and sauté them, stirring briskly for another 2 or 3 minutes. When the slices just begin to brown on the edges, add the garlic and continue cooking and stirring until the mushrooms are well browned and the garlic is cooked. Season the mushrooms with salt and pepper, and sprinkle with parsley. Serve on slices of hot Italian or French bread. *Serves 4 as appetizer; 2 as entree.*

GRZYBY ZE ŚMIETANĄ
(Mushrooms in Sour Cream)

1 *medium onion, chopped*	*salt and pepper to taste*
3 *tbs. butter*	1 *cup sour cream*
1 *lb. thickly sliced boletes*	8 *slices of rye bread, cut*
2 *tbs. flour*	*into squares*
2 *tbs. milk*	4 *tbs. chopped fresh dill*

Sauté the onion in the butter until soft. Add the mushrooms, and sauté for 4 minutes. Stir in the flour, and blend well. Add the milk, salt, and pepper, and cook, stirring, until thickened. Stir in the sour cream. Do not bring to a boil or the sour cream will curdle. Serve warm, spooned onto squares of rye bread and sprinkled liberally with chopped dill. *Serves 4.*

WHITE SAUCE FOR BOLETES

4 *cups of bolete caps and*	1 *cup chicken broth*
stems (if tender)	*salt and pepper to taste*
4 *tbs. butter*	1–2 *tsp. lemon juice*
3 *tbs. butter*	1 *egg yolk*
3 *tbs. flour*	1 *cup light cream*

Chop the boletes, and sauté them in 4 tablespoons of butter for several minutes. Drain them, saving the liquid, and set both mushrooms and liquid aside. Melt 3 tablespoons of butter, and stir in the flour, stirring constantly to avoid lumps. Add broth, the reserved mushroom liquid, salt, and pepper, and continue stirring until thickened. In separate bowl, add egg yolk and lemon juice to the cream. Beat together slightly. Add to cream sauce stirring constantly until cooked and well blended. Add the mushrooms to sauce, and serve over toast. *Serves 6 to 8.*

HEN OF THE WOODS   Like the sulphur shelf mushroom, the hen of the woods is excellent in casseroles, as shown by this recipe from Sally Benson of Nashua, New Hampshire, a New Hampshire Mycological Society member with a reputation for fine casseroles.

Don't be put off by the fact that the recipe includes a can of cream of mushroom soup among its ingredients. This may seem like carrying coals to Newcastle, but the result is very good.

HEN OF THE WOODS CASSEROLE

LAYER 1:

2 cups hen of the woods, sliced
¼ cup chicken bouillon

1 cup clam juice
½ tbs. unsalted butter

LAYER 2:

½ large onion, chopped
½ stick (2 oz.) butter or margarine

1½ cups seasoned bread crumbs

SAUCE:

1 can concentrated cream of mushroom soup
¼ cup milk

½ cup sour cream
½ can onion rings

To make the first layer, combine the first four ingredients in a saucepan over low heat. Set aside when heated through. To make the second layer, in a separate pan, sauté the onion in the butter or margarine until golden. Add the bread crumbs plus some broth from layer 1. In a greased casserole, alternate layers 1 and 2 until the ingredients run out. In a saucepan, whisk the last four ingredients together, heating the mixture while stirring. Pour the sauce over the layers, and top with the onion rings. Bake at 325° for 20 to 30 minutes. *Serves 4 to 6.*

CAULIFLOWER FUNGI These strongly aromatic mushrooms are very good when baked, fried in a batter, or combined in a quiche, as in this recipe from the Puget Sound Mycological Society's excellent cookbook *Wild Mushroom Recipes.*

SPARASSIS QUICHE

Rich pastry for a 10-inch pie
    pan
10 slices bacon, fried crisp
    and crumbled
1 cup grated Swiss cheese
1 cup sautéed Sparassis
    mushrooms

4 whole eggs
1¾ cups heavy cream
Pinch of nutmeg
½ tsp. salt
pepper to taste

Preheat the oven to 450°. Line the bottom of a pie pan with the pastry. Flute the edges. Sprinkle bacon, cheese, and sautéed mushrooms into the shell. Beat the eggs, cream, nutmeg, salt, and pepper together. Pour carefully into the pie shell. Place in a preheated oven. Reduce the heat to 400°. Bake for 12 minutes. Reduce the heat to 325°. Bake for 25 minutes more or until a knife inserted in the quiche comes out clean. Cut into wedges and serve hot. This is also good served cold. *Serves 6.*

SHAGGY-MANE   The mushroom has a rather mild though delicious flavor and may be prepared by adding cream to the mushrooms after they are sautéed, putting them in a soup, or combining them with cheese or eggs. Shaggy-manes are delicious when pickled. The cream of shaggy-mane soup presented below, one of the finest-tasting soups I know, is from that font of good recipes, *Wild Mushroom Recipes,* and the Coprinus Parmesan is from *Mushrooms of Colorado and Adjacent Areas* by Mary Hallock Wells and D. H. Mitchel.

CREAM OF SHAGGY-MANE SOUP

1 cup water
2 chicken bouillon cubes
1-inch cube of cheese
3 cups shaggy-manes, finely
    chopped

pepper to taste
2 tbs. butter
1 tbs. flour
3 cups milk

Add water to 2 quart kettle and heat. Dissolve bouillon cubes in the water. Cut cheese into small pieces. Add to water and stir until cheese is smooth. Add mushrooms and pepper. Simmer for about half an hour. In a saucepan melt the butter, and blend the flour with it. Add the roux to kettle and stir. Add the milk. Bring to boil for one minute to cook the flour. Serve hot. *Serves 4 to 6.*

COPRINUS PARMESAN

2 tbs. butter
1 egg
1 tbs. water
½ lb. firm, fresh shaggy-
    manes (large mush-
    rooms may be cut in
    smaller pieces)

½ cup Parmesan cheese,
    grated
2 tsp. dry orégano (more if
    fresh)
1 tbs. chopped parsley
garlic salt to taste

Melt the butter in a large skillet. Beat together the egg and water. Dip mushroom chunks in the egg mixture, and dredge lightly with cheese. Sauté the mushrooms over medium heat for about 10 minutes, turning them once until they are browned. Dust them lightly with orégano, parsley, and garlic salt. *Serves 2.*

OYSTER MUSHROOMS The oyster mushroom and its close counterpart *Pleurotus sapidus* fares best, according to many people, when cooked slowly with other ingredients in casseroles, soups, or in stews in crock pots. However, I have also stir-fried the oyster mushroom with vegetables with success. Two recipes are given below. The mock oyster stew is from Margaret Lewis of the Boston Mycological Club, and the second, a stir-fried recipe, is adapted from *Cooking With Exotic Mushrooms*, Kay Shimizu's interesting collection of recipes using various Oriental mushrooms.

MOCK OYSTER STEW

⅔ cup oyster mushrooms— 12 small tender mushroom caps or 6 large ones

1½ tbs. butter or margarine

3 to 4 okra pods, fresh or frozen

2 cups milk

dash of onion salt

salt and pepper to taste

sprinkle of mace (optional)

1 tsp. minced parsley

Simmer the mushrooms, cut oyster size, in butter or margarine for 20 minutes. Set aside. Frozen, sautéed mushrooms need only thawing. Drained, preserved mushrooms should be simmered in a little butter for 5 minutes. Slice the okra into ⅛-inch pieces and simmer in a covered saucepan in water to cover for 5 minutes or until tender. Set the okra and ⅓ cup of its liquid aside. Heat the milk in a double boiler (do not boil). Add the okra and the reserved liquid, the oyster mushrooms, a teaspoon of their butter juice, a dash of onion salt, salt and pepper, mace, and top with the chopped parsley. *Serves 4.*

OYSTER MUSHROOMS WITH BACON

3 bacon strips, diced in ¼-inch pieces

½ lb. oyster mushrooms, sliced

6 green onions in 2-inch lengths (use all)

salt and pepper to taste

MSG (optional)

dash of soy sauce

Fry the bacon until crisp. Drain off all but 1 tablespoon of fat. Add the mushrooms and onions. Stir-fry to coat, and sauté over medium heat for about 3 minutes. Add seasonings, stir, and serve. *Serves 4 as a vegetable side dish.*

Preserving Mushrooms

A time will come when the fortunate mushroom hunter discovers a mycological lode of morels, chanterelles, or other favorite mushrooms so plentiful that he or she will have plenty left over even after enjoying several repasts. One solution in dealing with surplus mushrooms is to preserve them. Depending on the species, the mushrooms may be dried, pickled, canned, or frozen.

Drying

Probably the oldest method of preserving mushrooms is by drying. It is also the simplest. When mushrooms are dried, the appearance and texture usually change, but the flavor remains. In some mushrooms such as the boletes, the flavor is greatly intensified. When drying mushrooms, it is important to evaporate the moisture from the mushrooms as efficiently as possible. Heat from the sun or another source is used to evaporate this moisture. Some mushrooms will dry quickly, others slowly.

One simple method is to spread the mushrooms out in the sun to dry. Larger caps are cut into smaller pieces about ¼ inch thick while the smaller caps are left intact. The mushrooms are spread on a paper bag in a single layer so that none of the mushrooms overlaps. The mushrooms are turned over periodically to obtain even drying. The mushrooms are dried when they are crisp and almost brittle, much reduced in size, and no longer spongy. The drying may take from one to three days.

My mother has been drying mushrooms this way for most of her seventy-plus young years. In my youth I remember seeing brown- or red-capped boletes spread out on a bag on a lawn chair in the back yard, wrinkling and shrinking as the sun's rays dried them. There was an earthy aroma when a piece of a bolete was held close to the nose. Since those days, by mother has gone a bit more modern. Before she places the boletes in the sun to dry, she now puts them in the oven briefly to kill any insect larvae that may be burrowing unseen in her mushrooms. She preheats the oven to 350° and then shuts the heat off before placing the mushrooms inside. After the oven has cooled, the mushrooms are taken out and placed outside. Although you may be tempted to dry mushrooms entirely in the oven, don't. The oven tends to cook and toughen the mushrooms during the time required to dry the mushrooms. Rapid evaporation, not heat, is the important factor in drying.

Even so, drying mushrooms can be an inside job; the mushrooms may be dried by placing them on a wire screen over a heat register, near a furnace, or next to a stove. The warm circulating air evaporates the moisture. Some people dry mushrooms on a string by threading the string through the caps and pieces and hanging them in a light, airy room or in the sun. To ensure even drying, the caps can be separated by a knot in the string or by inserting smaller pieces of mushrooms between the caps.

Mushrooms can also be dried efficiently with a simple dryer that you can build. Get a cardboard or wooden box at least 8 inches deep, remove the top, and line the inside with aluminum foil. Notch the top corner of the box and run an electric cord through it so that a 60-watt bulb can be placed inside the box. Put a screen on top of the box and your mushroom drier is ready to go. When the mushrooms are put on the screen, keep them

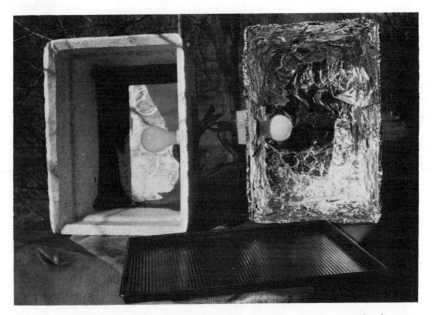

FIGURE 38. *A relatively simple mushroom drier can be made from a styrofoam ice chest by cutting a hole in one side large enough to accommodate an outlet. The chest may be lined with foil, as shown at right. The tray, in the foreground, which will hold the mushrooms to be dried, is placed on top of the chest.*

well separated so that air can flow around each one. A friend has constructed this mushroom drier, using a styrofoam container (ironically, its original use was as a cooler). Instead of notching a hole in the corner he cut a hole in the side of the styrofoam to nestle the socket for the light bulb. A tray was used to hold the mushrooms. The result of his efforts is shown in Figure 38.

Those of you who are not interested in building a drier can purchase a portable commercial food dehydrator. This compact, temperature-controlled unit has ten trays that can be used to dry mushrooms (as well as other foods). The dehydrator, which is a little more than a foot high, fits easily on any countertop in the kitchen or basement. Mushroomers who have tried this unit say that is is excellent for drying mushrooms.

Whatever method of drying you use, don't ever be tempted to use a clothes drier. One woman once tried to dry 5 pounds of the horn of plenty (*Craterellus cornucopioides*) by placing the mushrooms in a curtain bag. After poking holes in the bag for circulation, the woman placed the mushrooms in the drier. "The result," said the woman who shall remain nameless, "was one big fat dumpling. It took me a whole hour to clean the drier."

When mushrooms are dried the correct way (and I don't mean in a clothes drier), they should be stored in a dry place in tins, plastic containers, jars, or plastic bags. To prepare dried mushrooms for cooking, they should be soaked in warm water for about fifteen to twenty minutes. The time depends on the size and texture of the mushrooms. Any parts of the mushroom still hard after fifteen to twenty minutes probably won't become softer, and should be removed. Don't soak the mushrooms any longer than necessary; otherwise some of the flavor will go down the drain after the mushrooms are removed from the water. Some people save the liquid and use it in cooking. Once soft and pliable, the mushrooms can be used in recipes as if they were fresh mushrooms.

The premier mushroom for drying is the king bolete, or cèpe. It is the one dried mushroom that many great chefs prefer in making certain sauces. The bolete's nutty and sweet flavor completely transforms any dish to which it is added. Mushroom lovers go out of their way to visit Joes, a small restaurant in Reading, Pennsylvania, to sample wild mushroom dishes, especially Joe's mushroom soup. Joe Czarnecki, who has the only restaurant in the United States devoted to wild mushroom cookery, makes his soup from dried boletes. The recipe is reprinted below.

WILD MUSHROOM SOUP

2 oz. wild dried mushrooms, preferably Boletus edulis, soaked in water until soft	2 tbs. butter
	½ cup chopped onion
	¼ cup cornstarch
	salt to taste
5 cups beef broth	sour cream for garnish

After the mushrooms have been soaked, remove them from the liquid. Strain the liquid through a fine cloth and save. Slice the mushrooms, and place in a saucepan. Add 4 cups of beef broth and the strained mushroom liquid. Simmer for a few hours. Heat the butter in a skillet, and sauté the chopped onion in it, stirring frequently, until golden brown. Add the onion to the soup. Blend the cornstarch with the remaining cup of broth, and stir into the soup. Continue to simmer the soup until thickened slightly. Add salt, and serve. Use sour cream as a garnish. *Makes 4 to 6 servings.*

Freezing

Mushrooms can be frozen in several ways. You can simply cut the mushrooms into smaller pieces after cleaning, place them in freezer bags, and put in the freezer. Sulphur shelf mushrooms have been preserved in this way for a year, and the mushrooms are still good to eat. Or you can blanch the mushrooms for a few minutes before freezing. A third method is to sauté the mushroom in butter, margarine, or oil before freezing. After the mushrooms are cool, they are packed in air-tight containers and frozen. Some people freeze completely cooked mushroom dishes for later re-heating. Soups and sauces are good when frozen in this way. Partially dried mushrooms (slightly soft) can also be frozen in plastic bags and are very good when thawed.

Pickling

I first tried this delicious pickled-mushroom recipe at a regional foray when Greta Turchick, a New Jersey Mycological Society member, brought pickled inky caps for all to enjoy. The recipe can also be used to preserve other mushrooms such as the meadow mushroom.

PICKLED MUSHROOMS

Place a pound of mushrooms in a saucepan and cover with equal amounts of white vinegar and hot water. Bring the mixture to a boil and simmer for 5 minutes. Drain liquid from the mushrooms and allow to cool. Pack in a jar with the following:

¼ cup olive oil	2 cloves garlic, quartered
2 tsp. salt	1 tsp. mace
1 tsp. peppercorns	1 tsp. orégano

Cover all with white vinegar diluted with water. Cap jar, and store in refrigerator for two days before using.

Canning

Wild mushrooms canned in a pressure cooker have a lot more flavor than the canned mushrooms found on the grocer's shelves. Canning also preserves the shape and texture of most mushrooms. Because mushrooms are a low-acid food, they must always be canned in a pressure cooker. Make sure that you use only young, fresh, insect-free mushrooms.

The U.S. Department of Agriculture (Home and Garden Bulletin Number 8) recommends the following method for canning mushrooms.

(1) After the mushrooms are cleaned, cut the large ones in halves or quarters. Leave small mushrooms whole.

(2) Place the mushrooms in a saucepan, and add boiling water. Bring to boil again, and cover for about four minutes. (An alternative method is to heat the mushrooms gently in a covered saucepan for 15 minutes without adding any liquid.)

(3) In sterilized glass jars, pack mushrooms to within ½ inch of the jar top. *Important:* Use only ½-pint or 1-pint jars. Larger jars would require too long for the mushrooms to cook.

(4) Add ½ teaspoon of salt and ⅛ teaspoon of crystalline ascorbic acid to pint jars (half that amount for ½-pint jars). The ascorbic acid helps preserve the mushroom's color.

(5) Cover the mushrooms with boiling water, leaving about ½-inch space at the top of the jar. Run a silver knife down the sides of the jar to remove air bubbles.

(6) Adjust the jar lids, and process both ½-pint and 1-pint jars in a pressure cooker for a half hour at 10 pounds of pressure. Let the gauge return to zero. Remove the cover and let the jars stand until all bubbling has stopped. That's all.

Which Mushrooms to Preserve in Which Way

Which method of preservation is best for a particular species of mushroom? How will various methods of preservation affect the taste? Opinions vary, of course, but I consider Margaret Lewis of the Boston Mycological Club an expert on the subject. Having sat through many of her mushroom cooking demonstrations, and having sampled many of her excellent creations, I defer to her recommendations when it comes to preserving mushrooms, especially since she has also incorporated the opinions of others well versed in mycophagy. Her recommendations, reprinted below with her permission, are adapted from an article that originally appeared in the Boston Mycological Club's *Bulletin*. Some people may not agree with some of Margaret's opinions (some of her conclusions may even differ from conclusions that appear in this book), but Margaret's expertise must be recognized.

LONGEVITY OF TASTE AND TEXTURE
OF WILD MUSHROOMS AFTER STORAGE

MARGARET H. LEWIS

I fully expect to be laid low by all those mushroom cooks who think I've lost my taste buds, but this report is a result of forty years' experimentation. Influenced by members of the old guard [charter members of the Boston Mycological Club!], instructed by learned club associates, and trained to follow in the footsteps of our European-born friends of splendid culinary art, I've learned a few tricks about preserving mushroom flavor. So will you. Neither seasoning nor recipes are mentioned. This records only the taste and texture when stored mushrooms are first removed from bottle, crock, jar, and freezer.

If you've had better luck, I'll listen, but it's cheating if you sprinkle Instant Imitation Mushroom Salt on a dish when no one is looking.

SPRING

MORELS. *Morchella* (*esculenta, deliciosa*), almost forever good, do have their day. Broth made from any specimens tends to be delicious. Dried morels store long and well and stay fragrant in covered jars; though some are chewy after reconstituting. Sautéed frozen, morels are better than frozen raw, but the latter's broth has exquisite essence. Browned in chafing dish or baked stuffed in oven, they stay tantalizing in aroma. I've never counted the time of their lasting quality. They are best when dried slowly.

SUMMER

CHANTERELLES. *Cantharellus cibarius* (golden chanterelle), boiled to death, oversalted in crocks, dried to chalk, and frozen to a soggy state, have at last been plunked into the freezer uncooked, (or barely sautéed) to emerge a year later in a far more satisfying state, with aroma rather elusive. In six months, the dried may become too strong, the salted overpowering, the canned wishy-washy at once! Chanterelle flavor varies from year to year.

Craterellus cornucopioides (horn of plenty), frozen raw, keeps shape, flavor, very slowly leaving at year's end. Sautéed and frozen, it's limp, but tasty longer. Dried, it turns out mild.

SULPHUR SHELF. *Polyporous sulphureus* does not respond well to drying. If freezing, sauté to retain a better flavor, else salt it a little for later marinating within a few months, but cut into small pieces first. This velvety soft fungus' perfect state is in a rush to leave. Flavor won't last at all in canning. *Polyporus sulphureus*, dried slightly, but still in a pliant state, can be frozen as is without becoming chalky.

TOOTHY FUNGI. *Dentinum repandum*, sliced thin, dries well, and even smells inviting after one or two years, though only odor is left. Use crushed for spicy flavoring within a year, *Hericium coralloides*, frozen, sautéed, loses its lovely essence in a few months.

MEADOW MUSHROOM. The delicate taste of *Agaricus campestris* dissipates quickly. Freeze sautéed to avoid mushiness. Use within a few months. *Agaricus rodmani (bitorquis)*, a large agaric, becomes rubbery in age, but much less so in canning. If your tongue tells you they're good, you're starving.

BOLETES. Boletes, with sweet and nutty flavors, retain their savory ways and are worth every minute spent saving them for winter use. Sliced thin, most dry exceptionally well, though in a few years will produce that pungent odor and strong taste common to a great many mushrooms stored too long. Even *Boletus edulis* loses its famed aroma. Strangely, June's *Leccinum scabrum* has more flavor than late summer's. Expect it to be excellent dried for a year, as is *B. (Leccinum) aurantiacum*. Some boletes, when sautéed and frozen, stayed delectable even longer, but drying gives best results. Of boletes—*brevipes, chromapes, granulatus, indecisus, luteus,* and *rubro-punctus*—all held flavor well. Not so *bicolor. (Suillus* understood for some species.)

PUFFBALLS. *Calvatia (craniformis, cyathiformis, gigantea)* dried, either powdered or sliced, last a year, but are bland. Frozen and sautéed, a bit tasteless, they go in a year. They're tastiest in a sweet pickle, but disintegrate if kept a long while.

FALL

HEN OF THE WOODS. *Polyporus frondosus,* a favorite because it lasts a long time when canned or pickled, keeps its crispness, good texture, and pleasant taste. Not good dried. If frozen sautéed, taste is undefinable.

CAULIFLOWER MUSHROOM. *Sparassis crispa* stays crisp in canning— light flavor soon disappearing. Good almost a year. (Also applies to *Sparassis radicata.*)

SHAGGY MANE MUSHROOM. *Corprinus* demands quick action in the kitchen, but keep your fingers crossed. Count on the shaggy manes to make it, in either pickling or canning. If you have the magic touch, they'll also freeze, sautéed slightly or uncooked—but use before the year's out. They'll stay white too.

OYSTER MUSHROOMS. *Pleurotus ostreatus,* avidly sought, demands a tender state for canning. Though of little flavor, it's a splendid extender for dishes and lends itself to all kinds of cooking. Keeps well for a long, long time. In drying, it gets rather tough. Dry well before sautéing and freezing to avoid flabby texture when refrying. This applies to *Pleurotus sapidus* too. *Pleurotus ulmarius,* a tougher species, is not as useful.

Stalking Wild
(and Not So Wild)
Mushrooms in Stores

Contrary to popular belief, an American shopper is not limited to the familiar white supermarket mushroom *Agaricus bisporus* or its varieties. More than a dozen different kinds of mushrooms and other fungi can be found in supermarkets, specialty shops, stores in ethnic neighborhoods, gourmet sections of department stores, or they can be ordered by mail. You can, for example, eat prized boletes from Poland, golden chanterelles from Switzerland, delicious morels from Germany, truffles from France, the exotic wood ear or straw mushroom from China, and the highly flavored shiitake or matsutake from Japan. The mushrooms come dried in packages, canned, and, in several cases, are even fresh.

Although all of these fungi (with the exception of the fresh mushrooms) can be ordered by mail (see Appendix B, p. 271), I prefer to visit stores in the various ethnic neighborhoods to capture the flavor of the countries these people came from as well as to savor the flavor of the mushrooms. The phrase "you are what you eat" is true whether you visit the Chinatown sections in San Francisco or New York, the historic Italian North End in Boston, the Polish enclave in Chicago, or the German district in Milwaukee.

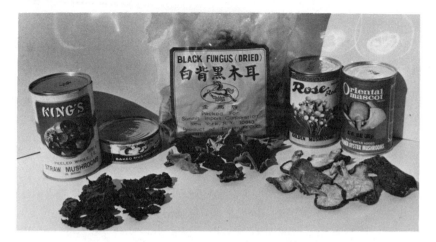

FIGURE 39. *Mushrooms available in Oriental stores. In the back row (left to right) are straw mushrooms, canned matsutake, black fungus (cloud ear), golden mushrooms (enokitake), and oyster mushrooms. The dried mushrooms in the foreground are (left to right) wood ears, cloud ears, and shiitake.*

Mushrooms from the Orient

A grocery store in Chinatown dramatically illustrates why Chinese cuisine is considered one of the finest in the world. It also reflects the important role of fungi in Chinese gastronomy. In addition to shelves and bins containing the leafy bok choy, water chestnuts, the crackling Peking duck, and other representatives of Chinese food, one can see dried or canned mushrooms (Figure 39). Labels on the packages or cans depict about 10 kinds of mushrooms, including the straw mushroom, the abalone and oyster mushrooms, the crunchy wood and cloud ears that are added to Chinese dishes for texture, and the shiitake or hoang me, as the Chinese call this fungus, one of the finest edible mushrooms.

STRAW MUSHROOM. The straw mushroom is believed to be one of the earliest mushrooms cultivated. The mushroom (*Volvariella volvacea*), as the name suggests, grows on straw. The straw mushroom has a gray to brown cap and a stem that grows out of a cuplike base. It is imported dried or canned into the United States from Taiwan. The straw mushroom "is as commonly used in Chinese and Southeast Asian dishes as the white mushroom [is] in Western dishes," says Shu Ting-chang in *The Chinese Mushroom*. (The title of the book refers to the straw mushroom.) The mushroom is very tasty, is excellent in steamed Chinese dishes, and can also be added to various stir-fried foods. The idea for cultivating the straw mushroom probably evolved when someone observed that the fungi appeared on leftover straw from a rice mill. Today, it is now widely grown on beds of soaked rice straw and cotton wastes, and is cultivated in China, Japan, Thailand, Burma, Malaysia, and the Philippines. The mushroom fruits rapidly, appearing within a week or two after the straw has been inoculated with spawn. "No other cultivated mushroom produces a crop in so short a time," notes Dr. Shu. The mushrooms are canned shortly after the cap emerges from the sheath at the base of the stipe. While some mushrooms lose much of their taste when they are canned, the straw mushroom retains an excellent flavor and is my favorite canned mushroom. I have talked with Chinese immigrants who have eaten the mushroom fresh, and they claim that the fresh straw mushroom is even more delicious than the canned variety, which is hard to imagine. This delectable mushroom is also called the paddy straw mushroom, padi straw mushroom, or Chinese mushroom.

SHIITAKE. A mushroom cultivated and eaten in the Orient that surpasses even the straw mushroom in popularity is the shiitake. Both the Chinese and the Japanese claim the shiitake as an important part of their cuisine. Today, the shiitake or hoang me is the second most important mushroom in world commerce, ranking behind only the cultivated *Agaricus bisporus* in importance. In 1975, about 132,000 tons of shiitake were cultivated for local use and export.

Early records show that the Chinese favored mushrooms during the Chou dynasty about three thousand years ago, and it is very likely that the shiitake was one of these. Over the centuries, this mushroom has been a favorite of royalty, the wealthy, and warriors. The shiitake was so coveted that people fought over the mushroom, and areas where the mushroom grew were kept secret. The mushroom was supposed to be not only extremely tasty, but also very healthy. During the Ming dynasty (1368–1644), a famous doctor, Wu Ming, called the mushroom "the elixir of life." The mushroom was believed to keep people vigorous and young. When prepared as a tea or extract, shiitake was reputed to cure various ailments. Recent research in the United States and Japan seems to lend credence to some of the claims. Kenneth Cochran, a virus researcher from the University of Michigan, has discovered a substance in shiitake that seems to stimulate the production of antibodies that help ward off invading viruses such as the flu. Another substance, called *lentinacin*, has been isolated from shiitake and was found to be effective in lowering cholesterol levels in the blood. The substance was uncovered by Japanese scientists I. Chibata and F. Tokita and reported in the scientific journals *Experimentia* and the *Journal of the Japanese Society of Food and Nutrition*.

The shiitake (*Lentinus edodes*) grows wild most frequently on evergreen oak trees that crown the mountain tops of Asia. The Japanese word for oak is *shii*, and the word *take* means "fungus"; hence, the name *shiitake*. The mushroom has a brown cap, pure white gills, and grows outward from the tree on a thick stem. In Japan, logs from oak and other trees are soaked for several days and then stacked almost vertically in rows in a shady part of a forest. The logs are then inoculated by painting spores soaked in water on the surface or by drilling holes in the logs and inserting wedges of wood containing shiitake mycelia into the holes. It takes about two years for the mushrooms to fruit. Recently, Henry Mee, a Shanghai-born scientist who founded the Kinoko Company in Oakland, California, a firm that has helped pioneer the cultivation of various species of mushrooms in the United States, has patented a technique that greatly reduces the time it takes for the shiitake to grow. With total environmental control in his indoor mushroom "farm," Dr. Mee can grow shiitake on artificial logs in forty-five days. (See "Growing Your Own Mushrooms," p. 245, for information on how you can grow the shiitake and several other mushrooms from kits in your own home.)

As a result fresh shiitake is now available in West Coast stores supplied not only by the Kinoko Company but by other California commercial growers. The availability of fresh shiitake is a first for a country that for many years had to be content with dried specimens from Japan. In the Washington, D.C., area, fresh shiitake has also become available in certain restaurants, because a Maryland farmer recently has been successfully growing the mushrooms outdoors on oak logs. Using the ancient technique of inserting wood chips impregnated with mycelia in holes drilled in the logs, Stuart Carr, working with Byong W. Yoo, has been able to harvest about 140 pounds of shiitake a year from his logs. The demand for these mushrooms has been so great that restaurants are buying all Carr can produce at $2.50 a pound, whch is a bargain for these prized mushrooms.

Fresh shiitake has made an appearance in another eastern city, New York. These shiitake, sold in specialty shops at $7 or more a pound, are being grown by a California firm, Gourmet Mushrooms Inc., and shipped to New York fresh. The mushrooms are cultivated on oak logs in a building with a controlled environment.

Even when dried, the shiitake has a very intense flavor and aroma. Only a few shiitake are needed in a recipe to impart a distinctive flavor. When lightly sautéed in butter, the taste and meaty texture remind some people of an exotic blend of filet mignon and lobster tail with a subtle hint of mushroom taste. I find it difficult to describe the flavor of many mushrooms, including the shiitake, for the tastes of fungi are frequently unique and have no equivalent among other food flavors. A simple descriptive word that still means a lot—"delicious"—should suffice.

The shiitake has twice as much protein as the common *Agaricus bisporus* and is unusually rich in calcium, phosphorus, iron, and vitamin D_2. Shiitake (hoang me) is used in various Chinese dishes such as soups, stews, or with pork or beef. A culinary feature of many Chinese banquets is the simple yet delicious dish containing a combination of bamboo shoots, water chestnuts, and hoang me. For those who like Japanese sukiyaki and tempura dishes, those dark objects among the meat and vegetables that contribute so much to the flavor of the dish are shiitake.

Formerly, dried shiitake was confined primarily to the shelves of Chinese and other Oriental stores. Now, they are appearing in gourmet specialty shops and in supermarkets in various parts of the country where no Oriental population exists. Dried shiitake are usually packaged in small transparent bags labeled forest mushrooms, black mushrooms, black forest mushrooms, shiitake, or simply dried mushrooms from Japan. The mushrooms when dried have wrinkled dark caps about 1 inch or 2 in diameter. The flavor distilled in just one of these dried mushrooms is impressive. The dried mushrooms sell for about $3.50 for a 4-ounce package.

WOOD EAR.   I did not fully appreciate the role of texture in the enjoyment of food until I became deeply interested in Oriental cuisine. To the Chinese (and the Japanese) many elements enter into the experience of dining, including the flavor, aroma, color, and texture of food. Chinese chefs are almost unsurpassed in their ability to handle texture. They enjoy *smooth* sauces, *crisp* vegetables, and duck *crisp and crackling* on the outside yet *tender* inside. Many Chinese delicacies may be either tasteless, colorless, or odorless, yet they are valued for the texture that they contribute to a meal. An excellent example is the wood ear mushroom.

The wood ear (*Auricularia polytricha*) is aptly named. The flat, brown, wrinkled fungus that is about as thin as a dime grows on wood, and, by stretching the imagination a bit, the fungus does look like an ear. A similar edible species (*Auricularia auricula*) grows in the United States and is collected by amateurs. In China, the wood ear is collected in the wild and also cultivated on logs. Hundreds of these earlike mushrooms may festoon one log. When fresh, the wood ear is brown and rubbery. Dried, it shrinks and becomes brittle. The mushroom is sold dried in bags in Oriental stores. When added to water, dried wood ears about the size of a half dollar may expand to five or six times their size in about fifteen minutes. The mushroom can also be grown from a kit containing a "log" inoculated with mushroom spawn. (See Appendix C, p. 273, for places where kits may be purchased.)

CLOUD EAR. The wood ear mushroom is often mistakenly grouped with another mushroom found on wood and sold dried in Chinese stores. The closely related mushroom is called the cloud ear or silver ear. Dried cloud ears are black on one side and have a silvery glint on the other side, caused by the reflection of light from hairs coating that side. This silvery glint accounts for the other name given to the mushroom—silver ear. It is also sold in this country under the name black fungus. According to Tak Wong, an amateur cultivator of mushrooms who grew up in China, the name cloud ear was given to the mushroom because it grew in a highland province northwest of Canton where the clouds seemed to scrape the hills.

The wood ear and cloud ear mushrooms are used in soups and in vegetable dishes to add texture. Either one is an important ingredient in the classic Szechuan hot-and-sour soup. The mushrooms can also be added to meat dishes. The Buddhists, with their vegetarian diet, have even used cloud ears as a sweet dessert, according to Cecilia Sun Yun Chiang in The Mandarin Way, preparing them by mixing the mushroom with equal amounts of granulated sugar.

SNOW FUNGUS. This white fungus is widely cultivated in Taiwan and Japan and is now being introduced to the United States. The Chinese prepare a sweet soup or a hot punch by adding the fungus to pineapple or other fruit juice. The fungus (Tremella fuciformis) is largely consumed for its claimed medicinal benefits. Other names for this fungus are white jelly and jelly fungus, because when wet, the fungus expands and becomes jelly-like. Tremella, the Latin name for this group of jelly-like fungi, means "trembling." The snow fungus is now being produced commercially in this country by Yamauchi Farm in Coyote, California. Japanese call the snow fungus shirokikurage.

OYSTER MUSHROOM. This mushroom is gradually becoming one of the world's most widely cultivated mushroom, although it still does not compete with such giants as the Agaricus bisporus and the shiitake. The oyster mushroom (Pleurotus ostreatus) is now cultivated in Taiwan, Japan, Europe, Australia, Canada, and the United States. Many amateurs are also growing this mushroom.

Canned oyster mushrooms are imported in the United States from Taiwan, but fresh mushrooms are becoming increasingly available. Some amateur growers sell oyster mushrooms from their homes or through nearby grocery stores; larger growers on the West Coast distribute the mushrooms through supermarkets and other stores. The mushroom is good in casseroles, soups, and stews.

ABALONE MUSHROOM. The Chinese have recently added another mushroom to the list of fungi that can be purchased in the United States: the abalone mushroom (*Pleurotus cystidiosus*). It was named abalone because its texture when cooked is similar to that of the shellfish. The abalone mushroom is related to the oyster mushroom and grows wild in the United States. After finding the edible mushroom growing on decaying wood in the forests of Taiwan, Chinese scientists decided to cultivate the fungus. Today, it is a very popular mushroom on Taiwan, an important center for mushroom cultivation. Canned abalone mushroom is now exported to other countries, including the United States. I have tried the mushroom and found it rather bland. Like the oyster mushroom, it can be used in stir-fried dishes, stews, and casseroles.

ENOKITAKE, OR WINTER MUSHROOM. This mushroom is another favorite of the Japanese. The name *enokitake* means "mushroom of the huckberry tree" around which the fungus grows. Widely cultivated in Japan, this mushroom ranks second only to the shiitake in that country's mushroom production. The enokitake is grown in bottles in a mixture of sawdust and rice bran. Grown under these conditions, the mushrooms form long stems and a small cap when they emerge from the mouth of the bottle. The mushrooms smell of grapes and taste like radishes, according to one enokitake fan. They are slightly sweet and spongy, says another, and can be eaten raw, or cooked slightly in butter or oil. The Japanese use enokitake mushrooms in soups, sukiyaki, salads, and appetizers. Recently, American growers have begun to cultivate enokitake, and these fresh mushrooms are now appearing in markets in selected parts of the country. Enokitake can be grown from kits at home by amateurs. The canned mushroom is also exported to the United States from Taiwan under the name of golden mushrooms. In the United States, with our predilection for shortening everything, fresh enokitake is sold under the abbreviated name "enok" or "enoki."

The enokitake mushroom grows wild in the United States, but here amateur collectors call it the winter or Christmas mushroom because it can be found growing on elms and other trees in the winter. I have seen it growing abundantly during a thaw on New Year's day in cold New England. The wild mushroom looks a bit different from the cultivated enokitake. Unimpeded by a narrow bottle opening, the wild mushrooms are not as leggy as the commercial variety. The winter mushroom (*Flammulina velutipes*) has an attractive shiny reddish-yellow or brown cap with a velvety brown to black stipe about 2 inches long. The striking velvet characteristic of the stipe is the reason for its Latin name *velutipes*, which means "velvet feet."

NAMEKO.   In Japanese stores in the United States, canned mushrooms called nameko (*Pholiota nameko*) can be obtained. This mushroom, which fruits on wood, is apparently cultivated only in Japan, generally on blocks of wood. It fruits in the wild in late autumn. The mushroom is not as widely cultivated in Japan as the more popular shiitake and enokitake.

MATSUTAKE.   Another mushroom that is prized in Japan and available here canned is the matsutake, or pine mushroom. This brownish mushroom, with cracks on its cap and a ring on its stipe, grows wild on the ground under red pine. Known for its aroma and flavor, the pine mushroom can reach a huge size, with caps sometimes up to 10 inches across. For the Japanese, the fruiting of the matsutake in the fall is perhaps the most important gastronomical event of that season. When news of the appearance of the matsutake reaches the crowded city of Tokyo, many of the residents, including businessmen and factory and office workers, head for the red pine forests around Osaka and Kyoto to join the local population in the search for the delicious mushroom. Carrying rice, sake, and cooking pots with them into the woods, the Japanese cook the mushrooms on the spot. For the factory and office workers, the matsutake picnics are a special treat because the excursions are paid for by management.

The matsutake (*Armillaria matsutake*) was also widely collected in earlier centuries. In the woods around the old Japanese capital of Kyoto, this mushroom was the prize find of both poor and royalty during the one month in the fall when it fruited. The mushroom was eaten immediately or preserved by salting or drying. Today, much of the wild matsutake collected in government-owned forests is canned and exported. Fresh matsutake also finds its way to restaurants throughout Japan, appearing, for example, in sukiyaki, or marinated in soy sauce and sake and then grilled, or steamed with fish, chicken, and ginkgo nuts in small earthenware pots.

The love of the matsutake mushroom was brought across the Atlantic by Japanese immigrants who settled in the Pacific Northwest. There in the evergreen forests, the Japanese found a close relative of the matsutake, a brownish-white mushroom that they called the "white matsutake." The first Japanese American to find this delicacy in the old Douglas-fir forests may have been one of the workers in the sawmills of the Puget Sound Region. The mushroom is still collected by the millworker's descendants, and each year in the large Japanese-American community in Seattle, a contest is held to find the largest white matsutake (*Armillaria ponderosa*). The window of Sagamiya's confectionary shop on Seattle's South Main Street displays the brownish-white mycological contestants that compete for top honor. Specimens weighing 1 or 2 pounds are not infrequent, although one year, explained Terumitsu Kano, a contest official who also writes for the local Japanese daily newspaper, *North American Post*, "we had a mushroom that weighed in at four pounds." A trophy is awarded to the winner by the Japanese consulate general in Seattle. In addition to displaying the American matsutake, Sagamiya's shop also buys and sells the

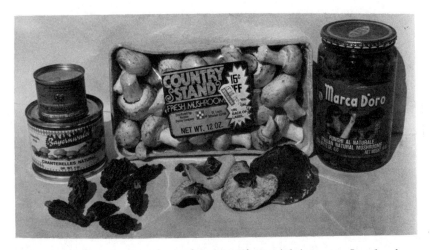

FIGURE 40. *Six species of mushrooms of special interest. In the foreground are dried morels and cèpes or king boletes. In the background (left to right) are canned chanterelles and truffles, fresh white mushrooms, and the Italian funghi al naturale (honey mushrooms). That tiny can containing about an ounce of truffles costs about $10.*

fresh mushroom for local consumption. Canned matsutake from Japan can be purchased in Japanese-American shops or purchased by mail.

Mushrooms of the Western World

Wild mushrooms are an important ingredient in the cuisines of many European countries. They include the by-now-familiar morels, chanterelles, and boletes, as well as the world-famous fungi, truffles, and other lesser-known mushrooms. Like the Oriental mushrooms, the so-called "European" mushrooms can be purchased in gourmet sections of supermarkets, in specialty shops, in ethnic neighborhoods, or by ordering through the mail. The mushrooms are most often canned or dried (Figure 40). Two commercial exceptions are the limited availability of fresh truffles in season plus the widespread availability of the champignon de Paris, or our familiar *Agaricus bisporus*. The dried and canned mushrooms are imported from a number of European countries including France, Switzerland, Poland, Germany, and Italy. In South America, Chile exports dried boletes to the United States.

MORELS. These mushrooms may be purchased dried or canned. Morels are not cultivated commercially. Instead they are cultivated in the wild in Europe, canned or dried, and then exported. Normally, French restaurants in the United States import dried morilles in huge plastic bags from France. Some canned products imported from Europe and sold as "round morels," "morel mushrooms," or "gyromitres au naturel" are actually false morels. At first glance, these mushrooms may look like true morels, but, as the label shows, these mushrooms have the typical brainlike folds of the false morels instead of a spongy cap. This mushroom, *Gyromitra esculenta*, is widely eaten in Europe, and is canned and exported to the United States. Although some people have become ill after eating large amounts of fresh false morels (see p. 27), I have not heard of any illnesses from the canned mushrooms.

CÈPE (KING BOLETE). Like the morel, the king bolete (cèpe, porcino, prawdziwy grzyb, steinpilz) is sold in this country canned or dried. The dried boletes are generally sold in 1-ounce packages for about $2. The dried boletes come from Poland, Yugoslavia, Romania, Hungary, Germany, and Italy, as well as from South America. For those who want to buy boletes in large quantities, canned boletes in 1-gallon cans are also sold. In the North End of Boston, almost in the shadow of the famous statue of Paul Revere in front of the Old North Church, Italian grocery stores display these one gallon cans of porcini in shop windows. The price: $100 a can. Smaller cans are also sold at a price more manageable to the pocketbook. A 10-ounce can of *Boletus edulis*, for example, sells for about $6. Of the two choices—canned or dried —most people including myself, prefer the dried. When dried, the taste of the king bolete is intensified.

CHANTERELLES. Beautiful golden chanterelles, with their fluted ribs, are also popular European mushrooms often seen fresh in the markets. They are also dried and canned. The chanterelles sold in the United States have been canned in water. The taste can be enlivened by sautéing them in garlic, butter, and parsley. U.S. shoppers may also purchase pickled chanterelles in jars. These mushrooms may be sold as "pickled yellow mushrooms," but the telltale picture of the trumpet-shaped mushroom of *Cantharellus cibarius* on the label gives away the identity of the chanterelles.

TRUFFLES. These are the "black diamonds" of French cuisine. Truffles may not be considered a mushroom by some, although they do have mycelia and a fruiting body that looks like a hard, dark earthball or a small black potato, and they grow underground. The truffle, however, is a fungus and a book on edible fungi that does not include truffles is like omitting wine from a French meal.

Truffles have been sought by humans at least since the time of the Romans. They are most familiar as an important ingredient in *pâté de foie gras*, although flecks of truffles are also used in cooking game, in sauces, and with scrambled eggs, to which they add an elegant taste. Dogs or pigs are trained as truffle hunters by French farmers and others to search for the "black diamonds." The truffles emit a fragrant odor strong enough to be detected by the animals, even though the truffle may be 8 inches underground. As soon as the dog or pig locates a truffle, its attention is quickly diverted with a reward of some other food while the farmer retrieves the truffle.

There are many different kinds of truffles, but the black truffle (*Tuber melanosporum*) of the Périgord region in France is considered the best. Another delicious truffle, the white truffle (*Tuber magnatum*), is collected in the Piedmont region in Italy. The black truffle grows in the ground generally under oaks, although it is also found under beech and hazelnut trees. Before World War I, the French ate or exported about 2,000 tons of truffles a year. Today the annual production has dropped to some 50 to 90 tons. The expensive method of searching for truffles and the fact that fewer black nuggets are found has sent the cost of the delicious morsels up to $135 a pound. In drier years, when fewer truffles fruit, the price of truffles in France rises to $250 a pound. In the

United States, a tiny 1½-ounce can of truffles costs nearly $30.

Only very thin slices of a truffle are needed to import a distinctive flavor to a meal. With the higher prices, however, the slice may become thinner or even absent from specially prepared dishes. Yet a recent event has gladdened gourmets and truffle fans. In 1978, the National Institute for Agronomic Research at Clermont Ferrand in central France announced that agricultural researchers Jean Grente and Gerard Chevalier had succeeded in cultivating the elusive truffle. Twenty truffles weighing a total of 2 pounds represented the first fruits of their efforts. Even though the first cultivated truffle had been produced in December, 1977, the scientists waited until they could produce another nineteen truffles before making their announcement several months later.

The researchers achieved their gastronomic breakthrough by inoculating trees with the mycelia of truffles. The scientists had known that the truffles form mycorrhizal relationships with the roots of oaks and other trees. The truffle mycelia benefit from nutrients supplied by the tree, while the tree flourishes in the presence of the truffle fungus. By inoculating young trees with mycelia carefully grown from spores under controlled conditions in the laboratory, the scientists were able to produce fruiting bodies of black truffles in about three to five years. The experiments seemed to show that not only can truffles be stimulated to grow with the help of humans, but they also seem to mature faster using this technique. Truffles normally take at least seven to ten years to develop. The technique has been patented and could eventually lead to a systematic method of truffle farming in France. Already, an organization called Agri-Truffe has been formed that sells and distributes seedlings inoculated with truffle mycorrhizae. More than 150,000 of these young trees have been sold.

The focus of interest on the truffle hunts of France and Italy (where the white truffle grows) has led many people to assume that truffles only grow in those regions and not in the United States. Yet they do. "We have more species of truffles in the United States than are to be found in Europe," says James Trappe, a U.S. Forest Service mycologist in Corvallis, Oregon, and one of the world's leading authority on truffles. Dr. Trappe even claims that some U.S truffles may be as good as the ones in Europe. "Among the West Coast species," he notes, "are three or four that look particularly promising for the table—and at least one that is equal to the European truffles." This one, *Tuber gibbosum*, is abundant in the Douglas-fir forests that extend from San Francisco northward to British Columbia. Food technologists are currently making comparative chemical analyses between the European and American truffles to confirm Dr. Trappe's conclusions.

Some Americans, whose appetite for European truffles matches those of truffle lovers in Europe, have imported truffle dogs from Europe in an attempt to find these elusive fungi in the United States. A San Francisco restaurant owner Adolph Motta brought a truffle dog from Italy and took it on walks in Sonoma County, California. Although no European truffles were found, the dog did successfully sniff out the *Tuber gibbosum*, which Dr. Trappe says is so good. Two other Californians, Henry Trione and J. Ralph Stone, have even more ambitious plans for uncovering truffles in America. These two Northern California bankers and a dozen friends have formed a corporation, Tristo Limited: Truffle Division, to find and sell native truffles. They feel that northern California has the same rolling terrain, moist climate, and limestone soil as those sections of France and Italy where truffles grow. The two men visited the truffle-growing regions in Europe, purchased two truffle dogs, and acquired access to 200,000 acres of land in California that seems promising truffle turf. The men have worked closely with Dr. Trappe and have hosted the First Annual California Truffle Congress. The two bankers have even designed a company coat of arms. The escutcheon is gold on a blue background and has four quadrants showing an oak tree, a truffle, a truffle dog, and a knife and fork. Unfortunately, Trione and Stone have thus far been unsuccessful in their efforts to uncover truffles with their dogs. Now they are focusing their efforts toward cultivating truffles in the United States by sponsoring a research project similar to that in France in which trees are inoculated with truffle mycelia.

Truffles can be purchased canned, or, if your pocketbook is capacious enough, you can have fresh truffles delivered in season direct to your home from Italy or France. The M. V. Wine Company in San Francisco can arrange to have fresh, whole black truffles sent by air directly from Paris. The supply is limited, and orders are filled on a first-come, first-served basis. A minimum of 1½ ounces must be ordered. The truffles remain fresh for two weeks after delivery. The prices vary, depending on the yield during the collecting season.

A New Jersey company, Paul A. Urbani Truffles, will import both the black and the Italian white truffles fresh from Europe for you. Urbani, the largest importer of white truffles in America, obtains his truffles from a large family estate in the Italian province of Umbria in the Piedmont Hills. He sells the truffles to various establishments, including restaurants and food shops. The European harvest begins in late September and ends in late November or early December; thus fresh truffles are only available in the United States during this period. The price of these fresh delicacies varies with the amount collected from year to year. During a dry season, as in 1976, when the "crop" was meager, fresh white truffles were selling in some New York food stores at prices ranging from $288 a pound to as high as $400 a pound. The black truffles are available in different grades and come whole or in pieces and peelings. The white truffles come whole in an "extra selected" grade.

The price per pound, though high, may also be somewhat misleading, because several truffles are needed to total a pound. And a thin slice from only one of these truffles is enough to flavor an entire tin of liver pâté. For those with a leaner budget, a smaller amount of truffles (1 to 2 ounces) may be purchased either fresh or in small cans at a more manageable price.

FUNGHI (CHIODINI AL NATURALE). This mushroom, which is sold canned in stores in Italian neighborhoods, does not have the fame of a cèpe or a morel, but it is very good. It grows commonly in both Italy and in the United States. The popular name for this fungus in the United States, the honey mushroom, is derived from the honey color of its cap. Each fall in our area, mushroomers search round stumps and trees for the honeys or *chiodini* as the Italians call them. The chiodini (*Armillariella mellea*) fruit in prodigious numbers, often blanketing a stump or ground around the base of a tree. Bushel baskets of these mushrooms are hauled out of the woods to be pickled and enjoyed later in the year. Bob Vitarelli, a second-generation Italian-American acquaintance of mine, vividly recalls seeing the bathtub in his house filled with honey mushrooms that were gathered by the family. The bathtub was a convenient storage area in which to clean and wash such large numbers of mushrooms before pickling them. During the chiodini season, the Vitarelli clan would gather to feast on a meal in which the star attraction was the honey mushroom. The dish varied from year to year. One year it might be veal with chiodini, another year spaghetti with a chiodini sauce.

The button stage of the honey mushroom is the most widely sought and collected among the Italians. This button stage is pictured on the cans and jars of chiodini imported into the United States from Europe. The mushrooms are usually labeled "Funghi al naturale," "Italian natural mushrooms," or "Funghi chiodini al naturale."

Despite the widespread popularity of the *Armillariella mellea* in this country, I have purposely omitted including this species in Part II of this book because it can too easily be confused by beginners with the deadly *Galerinas*, similar brown mushrooms that also grow on wood. Limit your collecting of chiodini to stores or mail-order catalogues selling Italian food products.

CULTIVATED MUSHROOM (CHAMPIGNON DE PARIS). The last "store mushroom" in this chapter is also one of the most familiar to Americans. *Agaricus bisporus* or *Agaricus A & Pensis* as mycological humorist and teacher Sam Ristich calls it. This chunky mushroom with the pink to brown gills is found in many guises in a store. Fresh buttons may be seen in baskets or paper cartons among the fresh vegetables. This mushroom may also be found on shelves in cans and jars, pickled, marinated, or in plain water. In the condiment section stand jars of these mushrooms powdered or in flakes for seasoning. Even freeze-dried *Agaricus bisporus* are appearing on the shelves.

Agaricus bisporus is the most popular cultivated mushroom in the world. Of the 661,000 tons of mushrooms cultivated in 1975, according to the U.S. Department of Agriculture, about 75 percent of this amount was *Agaricus bisporus*. The rest of the production included the shiitake, straw mushroom, oyster mushroom, wood ear, enokitake, truffles, and the snow fungus or shirokikurage.

The cultivated mushroom is believed to be a descendant of a wild mushroom that grew in Europe on manure heaps and other areas richly fertilized with manure. Although related to the meadow mushroom, this species differed microscopically (as well as in a few other ways) in having two spores attached to each club-like basidium, whereas the meadow mushroom had four spores on each one. Prior to the seventeenth century, people who wanted to eat this mushroom had to wait until late summer and early fall to gather the fungi in the wild. Then, in about 1650, N. deBonnefons, a Frenchman, noticed that the mushroom could be grown in a garden by casting pieces of the fungus and the water in which it was washed over an area containing partially decomposed stable manure. In his book, *The French Gardener*, deBonnefons said that such a mushroom "bed thus prepared, will produce you very good [mushrooms], and in short space [of time]." He added: "The same bed may serve you two, or three years."

Other Frenchmen readily accepted this idea, and soon mushroom beds began appearing in French gardens. In the next century, mushrooms were also grown extensively in the labyrinth of limestone caves beneath the city of Paris, where growing conditions were more uniform year round. The mushroom became known as the champignon de Paris, or mushroom of Paris.

The cultivation of this mushroom spread to England, the United States, and other countries. The mushroom was grown in caves, garden beds, greenhouses, and sheds. In the nineteenth century, the art of mushroom growing had progressed to a point where the mushrooms were now grown from *spawn*, which were dried chunks (bricks) or flakes of horse manure laced with the mycelia of the wild mushroom. When the spawn was added to beds, the mycelia in the spawn would spread into the surrounding soil. Eventually, mushrooms would spring up from the soil.

The spawn was supplied to the mushroom growers by spawn makers who collected mycelia from meadows richly fertilized with horse manure. In England, spawn makers would carefully monitor the fields each year, waiting for a prolific fruiting of the mushroom. As soon as one was spotted, the mycelium was dug up and rushed by train or lorry to be replanted in specially made beds of composted manure. The mycelium was then used to inoculate "bricks" of dried manure, which were sold as spawn to mushroom growers.

In the early 1900s, the practice of cultivating *Agaricus bisporus* in the United States was very limited. Commercial mushroom growing was largely confined to English, French, and Scandinavian gardeners who grew mushrooms under benches in greenhouses on estates in the New York and Philadelphia region. Then in 1905, a U.S. botanist, B. M. Duggar, perfected a technique for growing mushroom spawn that was to help vault the United States into its present position as one of the world's leading growers of the cultivated mushroom.

In Duggar's method, spawn was grown in the laboratory under sterile conditions from pieces of mushroom caps. The spawn that resulted was very reliable and could be mass produced. The new rapid method of producing spawn revolutionized the mushroom industry in the United States. More and more commercial growers began cultivating the mushroom. As more cultivated mushrooms became available, their popularity increased. Virtually all cultivated mushrooms now grown commercially in this country owe their beginnings to the technique developed by Duggar.

An important benefit of Duggar's technique is that scientists now had a way of guaranteeing that a particular strain or variety of mushroom that seemed ideal for commercial production could be propagated rapidly in the laboratory. Taking tissue from the cap of a desirable strain, spawn makers could easily grow mycelia of the mushroom. Today many strains of *Agaricus bisporus* exist, with caps that range in color from white to cream to brown. The white version is the most popular variety in the United States, although a darker-cap variety is preferred in some parts of the country, such as on the West Coast. The origin of most of the white mushrooms can be traced to a clump of pure white mushrooms that were discovered in a bed of cream-colored caps by a commercial grower in Downing, Pennsylvania, in 1926.

Until the 1970s, the mushroom growing centers in the United States were primarily located in Pennsylvania and, on a smaller scale, in other areas such as in California. Then in the mid-1970s, the mushroom industry "mushroomed." Giant industries such as Ralston Purina Company and Castle and Cooke, Inc. entered the mushroom-growing field, and soon modern facilities for mushroom cultivation appeared in such states as Florida, Tennessee, Texas, Connecticut, and Utah. Shoppers in Salt Lake City, Dallas and other cities formerly remote from mushroom-growing centers suddenly were able to purchase fresh mushrooms.

The consumption of mushrooms rose dramatically during this period. Before the growth spurt in the 1970s, each American was eating an average of half a pound of cultivated mushrooms a year. In 1977, the rate jumped to 2.2 pounds per person and is still climbing.

Today, the cultivation of *Agaricus bisporus* would stun de-Bonnefons. Mushrooms are now often grown in large, modern mushroom buildings covering several acres. Within these buildings, light, temperature, and other growing conditions are closely controlled. The cultivation process has also become highly mechanized. To give you a better idea of how a typical modern plant operates, let's visit the East Windsor Mushroom Company in East Windsor, Connecticut. The plant, built in 1977, is owned by the Castle and Cooke, Inc.

On the company's 80-acre mushroom farm, 50,000 to 60,000 pounds of mushrooms are harvested each month in a sprawling air-conditioned building. The mushrooms are grown in a large room containing rows of trays so high that a ladder is needed to reach the higher trays. The trays contain a compost made mostly of straw from racing stables. The bedding straw is actually a mixture of horse manure and straw.

When the bedding straw is brought to the plant, it must be changed to compost before the spawn is added. The bedding straw is mixed with other straw and is left outside in huge piles for fifteen days. During this period, microorganisms inside the pile become active in breaking down the pile. Much heat is generated by this process, temperatures may reach as high as 175 degrees Fahrenheit. Periodically, this pile is watered and turned over by machines. The composing material is then placed in large trays and brought inside to a room where it is cooked or pasteurized by its own heat and by steaming. The steam kills any disease-causing organisms inside the compost.

After the trays cool, they are placed on a conveyor belt and passs under a hopper that releases a controlled amount of spawn. The spawn is grown in bottles under sterile conditions in the company's West Coast lab in California, taken from the lab, placed on an evening flight, and flown across the country for use in Connecticut the next morning. A thin layer of peat moss, known as casing, is added to the surface of the compost. The trays are stacked in rows up to 10 feet high in a dark room where the temperature is kept at around 75° Fahrenheit. For the next few weeks, the mycelia spread throughout the compost. The room temperature is then lowered to 55° to 60°. In a few weeks, the first pinheads of mushroom buttons thrust through the surface. Several days later, the mushrooms may be large enough to harvest. Pickers with lights on their plastic helmets move between the rows of trays, picking the mushrooms and placing them in baskets. The baskets are taken to another room where they are mechanically sorted by size. The mushrooms are then placed in cartons or packaged in bulk and distributed by refrigerated trucks to markets nearby and to the New York City, Albany, and Boston areas.

Growing Your Own Mushrooms

Anyone can grow mushrooms in the home or outdoors without elaborate equipment. Depending on your inclination, you can have a wild-mushroom garden outdoors in the corner of your lot, grow cultivated mushrooms on your lawn, or raise several kinds of mushrooms in containers in your basement, living room, or even kitchen.

The different methods that amateurs use to cultivate mushrooms range from the dispersal of spores on the lawn to the cultivation of mushrooms from spawn placed in containers full of sawdust or other growing medium. Recently mushroom kits have been developed in which all the material has been put together for you. All you have to do is to periodically water a small log to induce fungi such as shiitake, enokitake, or oyster mushrooms to grow.

If you try cultivating mushrooms in your home, remember that fungi, like any other organisms, need the right conditions in which to grow. The correct temperature, moisture, and growth medium will vary from species to species. You, as an amateur cultivator, will act as midwife to the growth process, entering the process at any stage, depending on the method of cultivation you choose. Remember also that in nature, even when conditions may seem ideal, mushrooms may not always spring up in great profusion. By controlling these conditions, however, an amateur grower can increase the chances of success.

Growing Mushrooms from Spores

Some wild mushrooms may be grown by sowing spores. The spores themselves, caps containing the spores, or even water containing billions of spores may be used to propagate wild mushrooms in areas where the proper growth requirements exist. For example, if a mushroom species grows on logs, then the spores would be spread on logs. If a mushroom species is normally found in grassy areas, then the spores would be cast on the lawn.

According to Rolf Singer, when the shiitake mushroom was first cultivated on logs in China and Japan, new logs were placed next to the old logs on which the shiitake was already growing. The spores from these mushrooms would land on the new logs, and eventually shiitake would be seen emerging from mycelia that developed inside the new logs. Later, a more reliable technique was developed in which the shiitake caps were immersed in water. (Scientists today call this technique the *spore-emulsion method*.) Water containing billions of shiitake spores is poured over the log or sprayed over nicks cut into the wood with an ax. Mycelia then develop from many of the spores and form fruiting bodies. In inoculating new logs, some Oriental shiitake growers paint the spore-filled liquid on a log with a brush.

In the United States, various amateur mushroom growers have reported success in growing wild mushrooms using the spore-emulsion method. Oyster mushrooms, inky caps, and other edible mushrooms have been grown in this way. In *Wild Mushrooms of the Central Midwest*, Ansel Stubbs describes how he poured a dark liquid containing the black spores of the glistening inky caps (*Coprinus micaceus*) over a stump. Shortly thereafter, many fruitings of this mushroom sprang up. Harvests were then obtained for many years from this same stump.

When using the spore-emulsion method outdoors, there is

always the possibility that spores of other mushrooms are already present at the site where a species is to be cultivated. Once established, these spores produce a network of underground or underwood mycelia that makes it difficult for the spores cast by an amateur to get a mycelial hold. This problem can be minimized or solved for species growing on wood when new stumps or logs are used for the growing medium, because other fungi are not usually established on fresh wood.

Doug DeMaw, a Connecticut fancier of puffballs, claims that he can cultivate puffballs simply by sowing spores from the large mushroom on his lawn. After experimenting with various methods, DeMaw came up with the following technique. One or two puffballs that are dry and powdery inside are gathered from a field and placed in a paper bag. (A puffball that is powdery means that the mushroom is mature and is stuffed with billions of tiny spores.) The mushroom is then broken, spilling the spores into the bag. At various locations on a lawn, some dried animal manure is placed in the soil. (Bags of odorless dried manure are available in garden supply centers or hardware stores.) A few pinches of the puffball spore powder is sprinkled on top of the manure. About ⅛ inch of soil is then added on top of the seeded places and tamped down lightly to prevent the rain from washing the spores away.

The spores are planted early in the fall, to obtain a crop late the following summer. DeMaw claims that his technique works about 50 percent of the time and yields enough puffballs for immediate consumption and freezing for later use.

Mushrooms can also be grown from mushroom caps by emulating the sixteenth-century pioneer in mushroom cultivation, deBonnefons. Caps can be scattered (or buried) in the habitat preferred by the mushroom. Alexander Smith says that the beautiful blue blewits, an edible wild mushroom, can be grown on a compost pile or in a pit of old leaves by burying a few caps in the pile. The caps will inoculate the pile with spores, and "in a year or two," Smith says, "you will start getting a crop every fall." Foresters also encourage the growth of trees by mixing mushroom caps in the soil underneath the trees. The mushrooms used are those that are known to form mycorrhizal relationships with the trees. A common practice among foresters is to inoculate new stands of evergreen trees by mixing soil containing bolete mycelia from established evergreen plantations. Although the main purpose of the mycelia transplants is to encourage the growth of the evergreens (which it does), the luxuriant fruiting of edible boletes that also results underneath the canopy of evergreens is what interests the mycophagist. Some mycologists have suggested that a side industry of forest plantations could be the growth and cultivation of edible mushrooms such as boletes. This approach is already being taken in Japan with the matsutake mushroom in pine plantations.

You can grow your own boletes by matching the various species described in the bolete section to the trees in which they form mycorrhizal associations. Then transplant the mycelia and soil from the areas where they fruit to areas containing identical trees. This technique works best when the mycelia and soil are added to soil beneath young newly planted trees. It is less likely that other fungi have already become established under such trees.

I once removed some soil, caps, and mycelia of granulated boletes from underneath some established white pine trees several miles from my home. I then mixed the material in the soil underneath two young white pine trees that I had planted a few years earlier on my property. Before adding the bolete materials, no granulated boletes (*Suillus granulatus*) had been seen underneath the trees. Yet the following years, granulated boletes sprang up around the pines where the mycelia and caps had been added. Interestingly, no granulated bolete came up from another, nearby white pine on my property where I did not "plant" the granulated boletes. The two white pines receiving the bolete transfusion also grew better and looked healthier after the bolete transfusion.

Charles McIlvaine, co-author of the classic *One Thousand American Fungi*, also claims, based on his experiments, that the golden chanterelle "is also easy to transplant within congenial habitats, either by the mycelium or spores." The congenial habitats on which the spores or mycelia would be spread would be rich, leafy soil under hardwoods or under evergreens. To simplify matters, a chanterelle spawn is being developed at the Institute for Domestication of Wild Mushrooms in Europe that should be available soon for hobbyists.

Growing Mushrooms from Spawn Outdoors

Professional mushroom growers prefer to cultivate mushrooms directly from spawn because mycelia have already obtained a head start by growing in a favorable medium. When transplanted, the spawn will quickly spread if the conditions are right. In the United States, only three kinds of spawn are sold, those of the *Agaricus bisporus*, the oyster mushroom, and the shiitake mushroom. In Europe, an amateur mushroom grower has considerably more latitude. Spawn from nearly a dozen species of fungi can be purchased. They include not only the three species just mentioned, but enokitake, and the wood-inhabiting smoky-gilled *Hypholoma capnoides*, among others. Young trees impregnated with truffle mycelia can also be purchased.

Spawn can be used to grow mushrooms outdoors or indoors. In *Pilze im Garten* ("Mushrooms in the Garden"), an excellent summary on the status of amateur mushroom cultivation in Europe, Hellmut Steineck describes how amateurs can easily grow edible mushrooms from spawn outside on wood. Two methods that Steineck commonly uses to inoculate logs with spawn are a definite improvement over the time-honored spore-emulsion technique that many shiitake growers still use and are variations of another Japanese inoculation technique in which wedges of wood containing shiitake mycelia are inserted in holes drilled out of logs. In each of Steineck's methods, the spawn is sandwiched between a log and a chunk of wood that is temporarily cut out of the log. In the first method, a 2-inch-thick slice of wood is sawed off the top of a log 18 to 20 inches long. The slice is placed in a bucket of water while the log is stood on end. A border of sawdust is placed around the perimeter of the log, and the mushroom spawn is placed in the center. The bank of sawdust prevents the spawn from being blown away when the slice of wood is nailed back on top of the log. A nail is then hammered into the center of the wood to hold the slice in place. The log is then placed in the shade so it won't dry out. After the spawn mycelia migrate into the wood, mushrooms will later be seen sprouting from the surface.

In the second method, a wedge of wood about 1½ inches deep is sawed out of a freshly cut log and placed in water. The mushroom spawn is placed in the open cut, and sawdust is sprinkled along the edge. The wedge of wood is then nailed back in place. Aluminum foil is wrapped around the log several times where the incision was made. After three months, the mycelium in the spawn will have migrated into the wood, and the foil is then removed. Mushrooms will eventually appear on the log.

Almost any kind of freshly cut hardwood can be inoculated with mushroom spawn. Old wood is generally not used because the mycelia of other mushrooms may already be present. Steineck uses logs from trees that were cut down one to three months earlier. If the log has become too dry, it is soaked a day or two before inoculation. The mushroom spawn is inoculated in the log in the spring to give the mycelium time to grow.

The best results are obtained when poplar or birch wood is used. After three years, the nutrients in the wood are used up. Oak will yield mushrooms over a long period, although the mushroom harvest will be smaller. Cherry or beech logs are also widely inoculated, and an average five-year harvest is obtained from these logs. Many edible wood-inhabiting species, including the oyster mushroom that grows in Europe, have been cultivated in this way by amateurs.

Byong W. Yoo, a food technologist and Oriental vegetable farmer from College Park, Maryland, uses wood chips containing shiitake spawn imported from Japan to grow shiitake mushrooms on logs. Holes are drilled into oak logs felled in spring or fall, and the chips are inserted into the holes. If the logs are inoculated in the spring, the shiitake caps may begin appearing in the fall, although the initial yield will be small. "Optimum yield can be expected after about 18 months," says Dr. Yoo. The logs should be stacked in a shaded area such as a woodland or a roofed-over open area where air can circulate. The mushrooms appear in spring and fall; however, these mushrooms can be produced in other seasons if the logs are kept dry during the normal fruiting. For example, if you want shiitake in the summer, the logs should be soaked in water two two to four days, then stacked in an area where the temperature remains between 55° to 70° Fahrenheit. About a week after the soaking, the logs will produce fresh shiitake caps. A kit that includes 500 wood chips laced with shiitake spawn and a drill bit that matches the exact diameter of the wood chips can be ordered from Dr. Yoo (see Appendix C, p. 273). Thirty to fifty logs or about a cord of wood can be inoculated with these chips. A smaller shiitake inoculation kit with two hundred chips and a drill bit is also available. In 1974, in an experiment on Maryland farmer Stuart Carr's land, a cord of oak wood was inoculated with shiitake chips (procured from Dr. Yoo). The logs were left lying in the woods with no additional care. In 1976, about 110 pounds of shiitake were collected from these logs. In 1977, the output increased to 140 pounds. The harvest stayed about the same the following year, and the next two years Dr. Yoo expects "80 to 100 pounds before the logs deteriorate," which would bring the total harvest to at least 550 pounds!

An instant way of obtaining edible mushrooms from wood is to find a stump or log on which wild edible fungi are already growing and install it on your property. Water the log periodically to induce repeated fruitings of the mushrooms. This technique is commonly used in Europe. You can also transplant wood-inhabiting edible mushrooms by sawing one section of the log or stump containing the fruiting mycelia.

The log or log section can be part of a wild-mushroom garden. Logs containing oyster mushrooms, sulphur shelfs, or wood-inhabiting puffballs, for example, could be set at the edge of a woodland next to a grassy area containing meadow mushrooms. The logs might be moved to a wooded area where boletes are grown under evergreen trees. If you are easily embarrassed by the thought of passing motorists or neighbors eyeing you strangely when you are out watering a log with a watering can or hose, let the rains do the watering for you. This natural method of inducing fruiting has been successful for millions of years.

Growing mushrooms outdoors from spawn is not limited to just wood cultivation. In the United States, *Agaricus bisporus*, the mainstay of carefully controlled indoor commercial production, can also be grown from spawn in the "wild" outdoors beyond your doorstep. In addition to growing them in garden beds as was done years ago, several late nineteenth- and early twentieth-century books on mushroom cultivation also suggest a simple, carefree method of growing the cultivated *Agaricus bisporus* from spawn in fields, meadows, or lawns. In one method, a V- or T-shaped cut about 4 inches deep is made in the grass sod in late spring or about the middle of June. One side of the sod is raised, some soil is removed, and the spawn is inserted. The sod is then tamped down. "By cutting and raising the sod in this way," said William Falconer in *Mushrooms: How to Grow Them* (1918), the sod "is not as likely to die of drought in summer." The spawn can be planted about 6 feet apart. During the summer, the spawn will spread into the nearby soil. Then, if the weather conditions are right, a fruiting of cultivated mushrooms should result. To help ensure fruiting, some growers add compost or dried manure fertilizer to the hole before inserting the spawn.

The crop obtained depends chiefly on the weather. If the weather in late summer and early fall is too dry, don't expect much. A wet period after a fairly dry summer should yield abundant results. A good source for the spawn of the cultivated mushroom is the Mushroom Supply Company (see Appendix C, p. 273). The spawn is sold in quart containers.

Growing Mushrooms from Spawn Indoors

The cultivation of mushrooms does not have to be an outdoor hobby. It can also be a pleasurable "inside job." Amateurs in Europe and the United States have successfully grown several species of mushrooms indoors from spawn. The mushrooms, which include the oyster, *Agaricus bisporus*, enokitake, and others, may be grown in containers on shelves in the cellar, in closets, on windowsills, and in many other areas of the home.

When cultivating mushrooms from spawn indoors, various growth materials are used, ranging from straw, oats, sawdust, and rye grain to a mixture of peat and richly fertilized soil. The growth media or compost can be purchased ready for mixing with the spawn from mushroom supply houses. If an amateur wishes to collect his or her own growth material, it must be sterilized to kill any pests or molds that could contaminate the medium. The compost from a supply house is already sterilized. I use a pressure cooker (the large type that is used to can food) to sterilize the sawdust or rye grain that I use for cultivating mushrooms in my home. When one considers the sterile conditions that prevail in professional laboratories where spawn is grown, or the cooking process required for mushroom compost for *Agaricus bisporus* on commercial mushroom farms, one wonders how fungi in the wild managed to multiply for millions of years without the help of humans!

Amateurs have borrowed a technique from the Japanese to grow enokitake mushrooms in the home. The mushroom is grown in glass jars or plastic bottles containing a mixture of 70 percent sawdust and 30 percent rye grain. A mixture of straw, sawdust, and rye grain may also be used. I use sawdust from wood cut on my property. The rye grain is obtained from a local farm and garden shop. A lumber yard is another good source for sawdust.

The bottles or jars containing the compost are capped, wrapped in aluminum foil, secured with string, and placed in the pressure cooker for 60 minutes. After the containers are sterilized, they are cooled until the compost mixture has reached room temperature. The enokitake spawn is then mixed with the compost, and the jar cover is put back on. The container is kept wrapped in foil for a few weeks at a temperature of about 75° Fahrenheit, so that the mycelia from the spawn can permeate the compost. The foil and cap are then removed and the jars are placed on a windowsill where there is good air circulation and light; direct sunlight

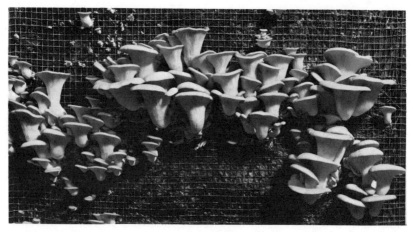

FIGURE 41. *Oyster mushrooms cultivated from straw in a vertical tray. Oyster mushroom spawn was mixed with the straw. The wire mesh holds the straw in place.*

however, should be avoided. In about two to three weeks, after periodic watering, clusters of enokitake will be seen sprouting from the jar openings.

Oyster mushrooms can be grown in a similar way. In one method, developed by Neil Anderson of the University of Minnesota, oats instead of rye grain are mixed with sawdust. Water is added to this mixture before it is sterilized. To make it easier to insert the spawn after sterilization, a 1-inch-wide wooden dowel is inserted in the center of the mixture. After the mixture has been sterilized and cooled, the dowel is removed and the spawn inserted in the space left by the dowel. This technique also reduces the chances of contamination because the jar is uncovered for such a short time.

The optimum temperature for the growth of the oyster mushroom is 75° Fahrenheit, although fruiting does occur at the lower temperature of 60°. A low level of light, such as artificial light from fluorescent bulbs or light from a north window, is needed to trigger fruiting.

The oyster mushroom, when it has been grown in a cylinder of sawdust and oats and removed from a jar, can be visually attractive. At a mushroom-tasting dinner of the Boston Mycological Club, someone once placed such a cylinder on the table. At first glance, many people thought that the white oyster mushrooms festooning the cylinder from which they grew were part of a delicate ceramic centerpiece.

Oyster mushrooms can also be grown on straw. In experiments at the U.S. Department of Agriculture's Western Regional Research Laboratory in Berkeley, California, R. H. Kurtzman, Jr., has successfully grown oyster mushrooms on pieces of straw that have been first soaked in very hot water (150°–180° Fahrenheit) for fifteen minutes. After rinsing the straw twice in fresh hot water to remove nutrients that favor the growth of other organisms, the straw is cooled in trays to about 75°. Spawn is then mixed in with the straw, which is then covered with plastic and left in the dark for about three weeks. The plastic is removed and nearby fluorescent lights are turned on. The tray is watered regularly to keep the straw moist. In about a week to ten days, oyster-mushroom pinheads begin forming, which develop into mature mushrooms. A light airy location is important for the oyster mushrooms, says Dr. Kurtzman; otherwise, the mushrooms will grow leggy.

To facilitate the proper circulation of air, Dr. Kurtzman grows oyster mushrooms on vertical surfaces by placing the straw in 6-inch-deep boxes (trays) set on their side. The trays are open at both ends. A wire mesh keeps the straw in place (Figure 41). The openings in the wire should be large enough so that the newly emerging caps can pass through readily. By having the trays open at both ends, the fruiting surface area is doubled.

This technique can be adapted by amateur growers. A tray, open at both ends, can be made by knocking out the top and bottom of a small wooden box or by removing the bottom from any solid container such as a plastic pail. The straw is added after it has been soaked in very hot water for fifteen minutes. Growing oyster mushrooms vertically not only encourages better circulation, but it also makes it easier to pick the mushrooms when they are mature.

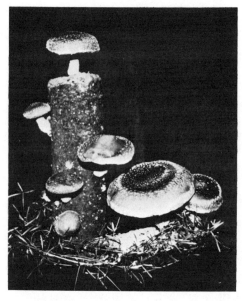

FIGURE 42. *Large brown caps of the shiitake mushroom grow from an artificial log. After the mushrooms emerge, the artificial log can be used as a decorative object, as shown here.*

Growing Mushrooms from Kits

Mushroom cultivation kits can be purchased in which everything is done for the amateur except the watering (Figure 42). The mycelia are already scattered throughout the growth medium and will grow and fruit soon after water is added. In 1976, Henry Mee, the same California scientist who developed the technique for quickly growing the Oriental shiitake mushroom commercially in the United States from artificial logs, introduced simple mushroom kits for five kinds of mushrooms: the wood ear, oyster mushroom, enokitake or velvet stem mushroom, the shiitake, and the *Agaricus bisporus*. Before then, only kits for growing the *Agaricus bisporus* were available.

The mushroom kits of the species other than *Agaricus bisporus* contain a small log that has been inoculated with mycelia of the mushroom. The 4- to 10-inch-high log is actually a compressed cylinder of sterilized compost containing sawdust, ground corn cobs, or peat. The log is first soaked in cool water for twenty-four hours. After the log is nailed upright on a wooden base, a perforated plastic bag that comes with the kit is placed over the log. The bag acts like a miniature greenhouse by keeping the log and air inside the bag moist.

The log and the inner walls of the "greenhouse" are periodically sprayed with water. A foam-rubber pad, placed under the log's wooden base, soaks up any excess water which may later evaporate, keeping the air inside the plastic bag moist. Depending on the species, the first pinhead-size mushrooms may appear from several days to six weeks later. The mushrooms mature in three to five days. Several periods of fruiting occur, and Dr. Mee claims that 2 pounds of shiitake mushrooms can be obtained from one log filled with shiitake mycelia.

The log is kept in any cool area out of direct sunlight. A corner of a room, the top of a desk or table, or even a shower stall (when not occupied) can be used.

In the mushroom kit for cultivated white mushrooms, a block of compost instead of a log is used. The compost is saturated with actively growing mycelia of the *Agaricus bisporus*. A bag of sterile soil (casing) that is spread over the compost block is also included. The mushrooms begin appearing about a month after you receive the kit. The mushrooms appear in flushes every seven to ten days. The first flush is heaviest, with successive crops becoming smaller as the nutrients in the compost are used up. Some mail-order companies will only ship *Agaricus bisporus* kits containing actively growing spawn during the cooler months. The mycelia may be affected and dry up in transit if such kits are sent during the summer.

In addition to Dr. Mee's Kinoko Company, mushroom kits for the oyster mushroom, shiitake, and perhaps additional species other than the *Agaricus bisporus* are now being produced by other companies in Europe and in the United States. A list of mail-order sources for the kits is given in Appendix C, pages 273–274.

Further Readings

This bibliography is arranged from the general to the specific. General field guides and other books on mushrooms are first given, followed by a listing of regional field guides and suggestions for more mycological wanderings among older but still interesting books. References for Part II are very selective. Only key research papers, reports, or books as up to date as possible are listed. Most of these references contain a bibliography that will lead you further into the subject. For the mycophagist who wants to delve further into more intriguing recipes for wild mushrooms, various mushroom cookbooks are suggested to augment recipes found in Part III of this book.

General Field Guides

BIGELOW, HOWARD E. *Mushroom Pocket Field Guide*. New York: Collier Macmillan, 1974. A brief, compact guide to 64 species of poisonous and edible mushrooms from the major groups of fungi.

LANGE, MORTON, and HORA, F. BAYARD. *A Guide to Mushrooms and Toadstools.* New York: Dutton, 1963. Although originally a guide to European mushrooms, this book is good for the United States because many species not found in other guidebooks are illustrated here.

McKENNY,MARGARET. *The Savory Wild Mushroom.* Rev. Daniel E. Stuntz. Seattle: University of Washington Press, 1971. Though written for the Pacific Northwest, many of the species are found in other parts of the country. Color plates are of poor quality.

MILLER, ORSON K., JR. *Mushrooms of North America.* New York: Dutton, 1972. The most comprehensive color guide (292 color plates) of North American mushrooms. Also available in paperback.

SMITH, ALEXANDER H. *The Mushroom Hunter's Field Guide.* Ann Arbor: University of Michigan Press, 1963. Describes 188 species; most valuable in the east.

General Books on Mushrooms

DICKINSON, COLIN, and LUCAS, JOHN. *The Encyclopedia of Mushrooms.* New York: Putnam, 1979.

KRIEGER, LOUIS C. C. *The Mushroom Handbook.* Reprint. New York: Dover, 1967.

PILAT, A. *Mushrooms and Other Fungi.* London: Nevill, 1961.

RAMSBOTTOM, JOHN. *Mushrooms and Toadstools.* London: Collins, 1953.

RINALDI, AUGUSTO, and TYNDALO, VASSILI. *The Complete Book of Mushrooms.* New York: Crown, 1974.

ROLFE, R. T., and ROLFE, F. W. *The Romance of the Fungus World.* Reprint. New York: Dover, 1974.

Old but Still Good

ATKINSON, GEORGE FRANCIS. *Mushrooms Edible, Poisonous, etc.* New York: Holt, 1911.

CHRISTENSEN, C. M. *Common Edible Mushrooms.* Minneapolis: University of Minnesota Press. 1943.

GIBSON, W. H. *Our Edible Toadstools and Mushrooms and How to Distinguish Them.* New York: Harper, 1895.

GUSSOW, H. T., and ODELL, W. S. *Mushrooms and Toadstools.* Ottawa: Dominion Experimental Farms, 1927.

HARD, MIRON ELISA. *Mushrooms: Edible and Otherwise.* Reprint. New York: Dover, 1976.

MCILVAINE, CHARLES, and MACADAM, ROBERT K. *One Thousand American Fungi.* Reprint. New York: Dover, 1973.

MARSHALL, NINA L. *The Mushroom Book.* New York: Doubleday, 1901.

POMERLEAU, RENE. *Mushrooms of Eastern Canada and the United States.* Montreal: Les Éditions Chantecler, 1951.

THOMAS, WILLIAM STURGIS. *Field Book of Common Mushrooms.* New York: Putnam, 1936.

Regional Guides

ARORA, DAVID. *Mushrooms Demystified.* Berkeley: Ten Speed Press, 1979. (A California guide.)

BANDONI, R. J., and SZCZAWINSKI, A. F. *Guide to Common Mushrooms of British Columbia.* Victoria, D.C.: Provincial Museum, 1976.

FERGUS, CHARLES L. *Some Common Edible and Poisonous Mushrooms of Pennsylvania.* Agricultural Experiment Station Bulletin 667. University Park, Pa.: The Pennsylvania State University, 1960.

GRAHAM, VERNE OVID. *Mushrooms of the Great Lakes Region.* Reprint. New York: Dover, 1974.

GROVES, J. WALTON. *Edible and Poisonous Mushrooms of Canada.* Ottawa: Canada Department of Agriculture, 1962.

HESLER, L. R. *Mushrooms of the Great Smokies.* Knoxville: University of Tennessee Press, 1960.

McKENNEY, MARGARET. *The Savory Wild Mushroom.* Rev. Daniel E. Stuntz. Seattle: University of Washington Press, 1971.

ORR, ROBERT T., and ORR, DOROTHY B. *Mushrooms of Western North America.* Berkeley: University of California Press, 1980.

————. *Mushrooms and Other Common Fungi of Southern California.* Berkeley: University of California Press, 1968.

SMITH, ALEXANDER H. *Field Guide to Western Mushrooms.* Ann Arbor: University of Michigan Press, 1975.

SMITH, ALEXANDER H., and SMITH, HELEN V. *Some Common Mushrooms of Michigan's Parks and Recreation Areas.* Special Publication No. 1. Ann Arbor: Michigan Botanical Club, 1963.

STUBBS, ANSEL HARTLEY. *Wild Mushrooms of the Central Midwest.* Lawrence: University Press of·Kansas, 1971.

WELLS, MARY HALLOCK, and MITCHEL, D. H. *Mushrooms of Colorado and Adjacent Areas.* Denver: Denver Museum of Natural History, 1966.

Part I Entering the World of Mushrooms

What Is a Mushroom?

INGOLD, C. T. *The Biology of Fungi.* London: Hutchinson Educational, 1961.

SMITH, A. H. *Mushrooms in Their Natural Habitats.* Portland, Ore.: Sawyers, 1949.

WENT, F. W., and STARK, N. "Mycorrhiza." *Bioscience* 18 (1968): 1035–1038.

WILDE, S. A. "Mycorrhizae and Tree Nutrition." *Bioscience* 18 (1968): 482–485.

Is It Edible or Poisonous?

AMMIRATI, JOSEPH F., THIERS, HARRY D., and HORGEN, PAUL A. "Amatoxin-containing Mushrooms: *Amanita Ocreata* and *A. phalloides* in *California*." *Mycologia* 69 (1977): 1095–1107.

BACK, KENNETH C., and PINKERTON, MILDRED K. *Toxicology and Pathology of Repeated Doses of Monomethylhydrazine in Monkeys.* AMRL-TR: 66–199. Wright-Patterson Air Force Base, Ohio: Aerospace Medical Research Laboratories, 1967.

COCHRAN, KENNETH W. "Interaction of Clitocybe clavipes and Alcohol." *McIlvainea* 3 (1978): 32–35.

DUFFY, THOMAS J., and VERGEER, PAUL P. *California Toxic Fungi.* San Francisco: Mycological Society of San Francisco, 1977.

HATFIELD, G. M., and SCHAUMBERG, J. P. "Isolation and Structural Studies of Coprine, the Disulfiram-like Constituent of *Coprinus atramentarius*." *Lloydia* 38 (1975): 489–496.

LINCOFF, GARY, and MITCHEL, D. H. *Toxic and Hallucinogenic Mushroom Poisoning.* New York: Van Nostrand Reinhold, 1977.

LITTEN, WALTER. "The Most Poisonous Mushrooms." *Scientific American* 231 (1975): 91–101.

RUMACK, BARRY H., and SALZMAN, EMANUEL. *Mushroom Poisoning: Diagnosis and Treatment.* Boca Raton: CRC Press, 1978.

SCHULTES, R., and HOFMANN, A. *The Botany and Chemistry of Hallucinogens.* Springfield, Ill.: Charles Thomas, 1973.

SIMONS, DONALD M. "The Mushroom Toxins." *Delaware Medical Journal* 43 (1971): 177–187.

WASSON, R. G. "Seeking the Magic Mushroom." *Life* 42 (1957): 100–120.

———. *Soma: Divine Mushroom of Immortality.* New York: Harcourt Brace Jovanovich, 1968.

American Mushroom Gatherers: Past and Present

GILMORE, MELVIN RANDOLPH. "Uses of Plants by the Indians of the Missouri River Region." *Thirty-third Annual Report, Bureau of American Ethnology* (1911–1912): 41–154.

PARKER, ARTHUR C. "Iroquois Use of Maize and Other Food Plants." *New York State Museum Bulletin* 144 (1910): 119 pp.

ROLFE, R. T., and ROLFE, F. W. *The Romance of the Fungus World.* Reprint. New York: Dover, 1974.

WASSON, R. G., and WASSON, V. P. *Mushrooms, Russia, and History,* 2 vols. New York: Pantheon, 1957.

YANOVSKY, ELIAS. *Food Plants of the North American Indians.* Washington: USDA Misc. Publ. 237, 1936.

ZELLER, S. M., and TOGASHI, K. "The American and Japanese Matsutakes." *Mycologia* 26 (1934): 544–558.

In Pursuit of Mushrooms
These additional guides will help you key out mushrooms.

GLICK, PHYLLIS, G. *The Mushroom Trail Guide.* New York: Holt, Rinehart and Winston, 1979.

MILLER, ORSON K., JR., and FARR, DAVID F. *An Index of the Common Fungi of North America.* Vaduz, Liechtenstein: J. Cramer, 1975. Lists common names and various Latin names given to mushrooms in popular mushroom guides published since 1897.

SMITH, HELEN V., and SMITH, ALEXANDER H. *The Non-gilled Fleshy Fungi.* Dubuque, Iowa: William C. Brown, 1973.

Part II Through the Year with Mushrooms

SPRING

Morel

BARTELLI, INGRID. *May Is Morel Month in Michigan.* Cooperative Extension Service Bulletin R-614. East Lansing: Michigan State University, no date.

SUMMER

Vase-shaped Mushroom

BIGELOW, H. E. "The Cantharelloid Fungi of New England and Adjacent Areas." *Mycologia* 70 (1978): 707–756.

CORNER, E. J. H. "A Monograph of Cantharelloid Fungi." *Ann. Bot. Mem.* 2 (1966): 1–255.

Sulphur Shelf Mushroom

OVERHOLTS, L. O. *The Polyporaceae of the United States, Alaska, and Canada.* Ann Arbor: University of Michigan Press, 1953.

Teeth Fungus

HARRISON, K. "The Genus Hericium in North America." *Michigan Botanist* 12 (1973): 177–194.

Meadow Mushroom and Rodman's Mushroom

KERRIGAN, RICK. "Poisonous Species in the Genus Agaricus." *Mycena News* 28 (1978): 46.

See also references for growing your own mushrooms on page 267.

Puffball

BENEKE, EVERETT S. "Calvatia, Calvacin, and Cancer." *Mycologia* 60 (1963): 257–270.

COKER, WILLIAM C., and COUCH, JOHN N. *The Gasteromycetes of the Eastern United States and Canada.* Reprint. New York: Dover, 1973.

ROLAND, J. F., *et al.* "Calvacin: A New Antitumor Agent." *Science* 132 (1960): 1897.

ROLFE, R. T., and ROLFE, F. W. *The Romance of the Fungus World.* New York: Dover, 1974. Chapter 7, pp. 127–147.

SMITH, ALEXANDER H. *Puffballs and Their Allies in Michigan.* Ann Arbor: University of Michigan Press, 1951.

FALL

Bolete

BARTELLI, INGRID. *Best of the Boletes.* Cooperative Extension Service Bulletin E-926. East Lansing: Michigan State University, no date.

BULLER, A. H. REGINALD. "Fungus Lore of the Greeks and Romans." *British Mycological Society Transactions* 5 (1914): 21–26.

COKER, WILLIAM CHAMBERS, and BEERS, ALMA HOLLAND. *The*

Boleti of North Carolina. Reprint. New York: Dover, 1973.

GRUND, D. W., and HARRISON, K. A. *Nova Scotian Boletes*. Vaduz, Liechtenstein: J. Cramer, 1976.

HOMOLA, RICHARD L., and MISTRETTA, PAUL A. *Ectomycorrhizae of Maine: A Listing of Boletaceae with the Associated Hosts*. Agricultural Experiment Station Bulletin 735. Orono: University of Maine, January, 1977.

SMITH, ALEXANDER H., and THIERS, HARRY D. *The Boletes of Michigan*. Ann Arbor: University of Michigan Press, 1971.

SNELL, WALTER H., and DICK, E. A. *The Boleti of Northeastern America*. Vaduz, Liechtenstein: J. Cramer, 1970.

THIERS, HARRY D. *California Mushrooms: A Field Guide to Boletes*. New York: Hafner, 1975.

Hen of the Woods and Many-capped Polypore
See general references at the beginning of bibliography.

Cauliflower Fungus and Curly Sparassis
MARTIN, K. J., and GILBERTSON, R. L. "Cultural and Other Morphological Studies of Sparassis radicata and Related Species." *Mycologia* 68 (1976): 622–639.

Shaggy-Mane
BARTELLI, INGRID. *Wood Waste Makes Wonderful Mushrooms*. Cooperative Extension Service Bulletin E-925. East Lansing: Michigan State University, no date.

BULLER, A. H. REGINALD. "Various Remarks on the Coprini." *Researches on Fungi* 4 (1931): 63–77.

HOUGHTON, W. "Notices of Fungi in Greek and Latin Authors." *Annals and Magazine of Natural History* Series 5, 15 (1885): 22–49.

Oyster, Lilac, and Angel Wings
ANDERSON, N. A., WANG, S. S., and SCHWANDT, J. W. "The Pleurotus ostreatus-sapidus Species Complex." *Mycologia* 65 (1973): 28–35.

BARTELLI, INGRID. *Mushrooms Grow on Stumps*. Cooperative Extension Service Bulletin E-924. East Lansing: Michigan State University, no date.

LAMBERT, EILEEN. "Oysters on Trees." *National Parks and Conservation Magazine* November, 1973, pp. 20–21.

Part III Mushrooms for the Table

PREPARING AND PRESERVING MUSHROOMS

COFFIN, GEORGE, and LEWIS, MARGARET. *Twenty Common Mushrooms and How to Cook Them.* Boston: International Pocket Library, 1965.

GRIGSON, JANE. *The Mushroom Feast.* New York: Knopf, 1975.

MYCOLOGICAL SOCIETY OF SAN FRANCISCO. *Kitchen Magic with Mushrooms.* San Francisco: Mycological Society of San Francisco, 1973.

NEW JERSEY MYCOLOGICAL ASSOCIATION. *Mycophagist's Corner.* Franklin: New Jersey Mycological Association, 1978.

PUGET SOUND MYCOLOGICAL SOCIETY. *Wild Mushroom Recipes.* Seattle: Pacific Search, 1973.

SHIMIZU, KAY. *Cooking with Exotic Mushrooms.* Tokyo: Shufunotomo, 1977.

STALKING WILD (AND NOT SO WILD) MUSHROOMS IN STORES

CHELMINSKI, RUDOLPH. "French Science Robs the Truffle of Its Gallic Romance and Its Rarity With the First Crop from a Greenhouse." *Horticulture,* May, 1978, pp. 15–19.

HOPSON, JANET L. "Truffles, the Bottom Link." *Science News,* October 18, 1975, pp. 250–251.

SHU TING-CHANG. *The Chinese Mushroom (Volvariella volvacea).* Hong Kong: The Chinese University of Hong Kong, 1972.

JAPANESE FOREST MUSHROOM PROMOTION ASSOCIATION. *The Japanese Forest Mushroom.* Tokyo: Japanese Forest Mushroom Promotion Association, no date.

JONG, S. C., and PENG, J. T. "Identity and Cultivation of a New Commercial Mushroom in Taiwan." *Mycologia* 67 (1975): 1235–1238.

RAMSBOTTOM, J. *Mushrooms and Toadstools.* London: Collins, 1953. Chapter 22, pp. 258–272.

GROWING YOUR OWN MUSHROOMS

ATKINS, F. C. *Mushroom Growing Today*. New York: Macmillan, 1966.

CHIU, R., et al. eds. *Mushroom Science IX (Part II)*. Proceedings of the IX International Scientific Congress on the Cultivation of Edible Fungi, Taipei, November, 1974. Taiwan: The Chinese Society for Horticultural Science, 1977.

DUGGAR, B. M. *Mushroom Growing*. New York: Orange Judd, 1920.

FALCONER, WILLIAM. *Mushrooms: How to Grow Them*. New York: Orange Judd, 1918.

KURTZMAN, RALPH. *Assorted Readings from Proceedings of Seminar on Mushroom Research and Production*. Karachi: Pakistan Press, 1975.

MORGAN, TOYA. "You Can Grow Your Own Mushrooms." *Flower and Garden*, September, 1977, pp. 48–50.

MUELLER, JO. *Growing Your Own Mushrooms*. Charlotte, Vt.: Garden Way Publishing, 1976.

SHU TING-CHANG, and HAYES, W. A. *Biology and Cultivation of Fungi*. New York: Academic Press, 1978.

SINGER, ROLF. *Mushrooms and Truffles*. New York: Interscience Publishers, 1961.

STEINECK, HELLMUT. *Pilze im Garten*. Stuttgart: Verlag Eugen Ulmer, 1976.

Amateur Mycological Societies in North America

CALIFORNIA

Mycological Society of
  San Francisco
P.O. Box 904
San Francisco, California 94101

Los Angeles Mycological Society
Los Angeles Museum of Natural
  History
c/o Botanical Curator
900 Exposition Boulevard
Los Angeles, California 90007

Humbolt Bay Mycological Society
c/o Ms. Pam Kessler
P.O. Box 75
Bayside, California 95524

COLORADO

Colorado Mycological Society
909 York Street
Denver, Colorado 80206

Pikes Peak Mycological Society
10565 Burgess Road
Colorado Springs, Colorado 80908

CONNECTICUT

Connecticut Mycological
  Association
Route 3
Box 137 B
Pound Ridge, New York 10576

Connecticut Valley Mycological
  Association
169 Edwards Road
Cheshire, Connecticut 06410

Nutmeg Mycological Society
P.O. Box 530
Groton, Connecticut 06340

DISTRICT OF COLUMBIA

Mycological Association of
  Washington, D.C.

6203 Westbrook Drive
New Carrollton, Maryland 20784

IDAHO

North Idaho Mycological
Association
Route No. 5
Box 186
Post Falls, Idaho 83854

Southern Idaho Mycological
Association
P.O. Box 843
Boise, Idaho 83701

ILLINOIS

Illinois Mycological Association
4744 South Kimbark Avenue
Chicago, Illinois 60615

LOUISIANA

New Orleans Mycological Society
c/o William Newman
722 Cherokee Street
New Orleans, Louisiana 70118

MASSACHUSETTS

Boston Mycological Club
16 Divinity Avenue
Cambridge, Massachusetts 02138

MINNESOTA

Minnesota Mycological Society
4744 Upton Avenue, South
Minneapolis, Minnesota 53410

NEW HAMPSHIRE

New Hampshire Mycological
Society
14 Brookline Street
Nashua, New Hampshire 03060

NEW JERSEY

New Jersey Mycological
Association
709 Reba Road
Landing, New Jersey 07850

NEW YORK

New York Mycological Society
c/o Ms. Stephanie Hawthorn
132 West Thirteenth Street
New York, New York 10011

Buffalo Mycological Society
Buffalo Museum of Science
Humboldt Parkway
Buffalo, New York 14211

Montauk Mushroom Club
57 Henry Street
Southampton, New York 11968

The Long Island Mycological Club
128 Audley Street
Kew Gardens, New York 11418

OHIO

North American Mycological
Association
4245 Redinger Road
Portsmouth, Ohio 45662

Ohio Mushroom Society
c/o Walter Sturgeon
121 Brookline Road
Youngstown, Ohio 44505

OREGON

Oregon Mycological Society
9515 North Pier Park Place
Portland, Oregon 97203

Oregon Coast Mycological Society
Otter Rock, Oregon 97369

TEXAS

Texas Mycological Society
c/o Dr. Cynthia A. Rogers
Houston Baptist University
7502 Fondren Road
Houston, Texas 77074

WASHINGTON

Puget Sound Mycological Society
200 Second Avenue North
Seattle, Washington 98109

Tacoma Mushroom Society
2207 North Washington
Tacoma, Washington 98406

Kitsap Peninsula Mycological
Society
P.O. Box 263
Bremerton, Washington 98310

Central Washington Mycological
Society
Box 2214
Yakima, Washington 98907

Wenatchee Valley Mushroom
Society
c/o Harold Larsen
419 Douglas Street
Wenatchee, Washington 98801

Twin Harbors Mushroom Club
Route 2
Box 193
Hoquiam, Washington 98550

Snohomish County Mycological
Society
12225 Thirteenth Drive, S.E.
Everett, Washington 98204

Spokane Mushroom Club
P.O. Box 2791
Spokane, Washington 99220

WISCONSIN

Wisconsin Mycological Society
3270 North Cambridge Avenue
Milwaukee, Wisconsin 53204

WYOMING

Lander Valley Mycological Society
Fremont County Library
451 North Second
Lander, Wyoming 82520

CANADA

Mycological Society of Toronto
239 Thirtieth Street
Toronto, Ontario
MW8 3C9

Cercle des Mycologues Amateur
de Quebec
Pavillon Comtois
Université Laval
Quebec
GIK 7P4

Mushrooms by Mail

If you live in an area containing large ethnic neighborhoods whose cultural tradition includes mushrooms, you can obtain various kinds of mushrooms simply by visiting these neighborhoods. Department stores in metropolitan areas often have food departments that specialize in unusual gourmet items, including mushrooms. Check also in the yellow pages under such subject headings as "Gourmet Shops," "Oriental Goods," and "Grocers, Retail"; in the latter case, their entries will often list their specialties.

You may also shop by mail at the establishments listed below. Most will send you a catalogue or price list.

ORIENTAL MUSHROOMS

Anzen Japanese Foods and Imports
736 Northeast Union Avenue
Portland, Oregon 79232

The Asian Express Co.
P.O. Box 375
Pelham, New York 10803

East Wind
2801 Broadway
New York, New York 10025

Gourmet Mushrooms, Inc.
P.O. Box 391
Sebastopol, California 95472

Katagiri and Co., Inc.
224 East Fifty-ninth Street
New York, New York 10022

Omura Japanese Food and
   Gift Shop
3811 Payne Avenue
Cleveland, Ohio 44114

Uwajimaya
Box 3003
Seattle, Washington 98114

Wing Fat Co.
33–35 Mott Street
New York, New York 10013

MUSHROOMS FROM THE WEST

Bremen House
200 East Eighty-sixth Street
New York, New York 10028

J. A. Demonchaux Co.
827 North Kansas Avenue
Topeka, Kansas 66608

Fauchon
26, Place de la Madeleine
75008, Paris 8ᵉ, France

Hediard
21, Place de la Madeleine
Paris 8ᵉ, France

Le Jardin du Gourmet
Les Echalottes
West Danville, Vermont 05873

Manganaro's
488 Ninth Avenue
New York, New York 10018

H. L. Roth & Son
Lekvar-by-the Barrel
1577 First Avenue
New York, New York 10028

Paul A. Urbani Truffles
P.O. Box 2054
Trenton, New Jersey 08607

M. V. Wine Company
576 Folsom Street
San Francisco, California 94105

Supply Sources for Growing Your Own Mushrooms

KITS

The Kinoko Company, P.O. Box 6425, Oakland, California 94621. Produces five kits: shiitake, wood ear, tree oyster (*Pleurotus ostreatus*), velvet stem (enokitake), and common button mushroom (*Agaricus bisporus*).

Oregon Mushroom & Food Co., Inc., Route 3, Box 204, Gresham, Oregon 97005. Produces Shimeji Garden Kits (*Pleurotus ostreatus*) for home growing in bottles.

Edmund Scientific Company, 7782 Edscorp Building, Barrington, New Jersey 08007. Kit for growing *Agaricus bisporus*.

River Valley Ranch, P.O. Box 898, New Munster, Wisconsin 53152. Kit for growing *Agaricus bisporus*.

Grow-your-own mushroom kits can also be purchased in many garden centers, department stores, and from nursery and seed catalogues. Some of these nursery and seed firms are:

Thompson & Morgan, Inc., P.O. Box 100, Farmingdale, New Jersey 07727.

Nichols Garden Nursery, 1190 North Pacific Highway, Albany, Oregon 97321.

Henry Field Seed and Nursery Company, 407 Sycamore Street, Shenandoah, Iowa 51601.

Mellinger's, 2310 West South Range, North Lima, Ohio 44452.

Gurney Seed & Nursery Co., 2nd and Capitol Streets, Yankton, South. Dakota 57079.

Lakeland Nurseries Sales, 340 Poplar Street, Hanover, Pennsylvania 17331.

SPAWN

OYSTER MUSHROOM

Somycel, U.S., Inc., Box 476, Avondale, Pennsylvania 19311.

The Kinoko Company, P.O. Box 6425, Oakland, California 94621.

SHIITAKE

Dr. Yoo Farm, P.O. Box 290, College Park, Maryland 20740. Supplies wood chips containing shiitake spawn to inoculate logs. Regular shiitake kit (500 shiitake spawn wood chips, 1 drill bit), $26.50. Small shiitake kit: (200 spawn chips, 1 drill bit), $13.50. Also, a booklet on growing shiitake, $2.50.

The Kinoko Company, P.O. Box 6425, Oakland, California 94621.

CULTIVATED STORE MUSHROOM (Agaricus bisporus)

Mushroom Supply Company, Toughkenamon, Pennsylvania 19374. An excellent source of spawn for amateurs. Spawn of the cultivated mushrooms comes in two types: dried or moist. Dried spawn, which is a crumbly mixture of inactive mycelia and growth media, will keep indefinitely, until ready to be used. Moist spawn, which is usually supplied to commercial growers, is mycelia actively growing on rice grain. It has to be shipped as rapidly as possible (which can be quite expensive) and must be used upon receipt. The dried spawn is recommended for beginners. It is sold by the quart ($3.50 a quart shipped anywhere east of the Mississippi, $3.75 west of the Mississippi).

The Kinoko Company, P.O. Box 6425, Oakland, California 94621. Sells Agaricus bisporus spawn as well as pasteurized compost in which to grow the spawn.

Seed and Garden Companies. These companies usually list this spawn in their catalogues, but it is generally more expensive than if you order the spawn direct from a company that produces the spawn.

ILLUSTRATION CREDITS

BLACK-AND-WHITE PHOTOGRAPHS

Donald M. Simons: 3; Alexander H. Smith and the University of Michigan Herbarium: 5, 9, 15; Cornell University Plant Pathology Herbarium: 6, 7, 18, 28, 32, 33; Emily Johnson: 13, 14; Howard E. Bigelow: 21, 23, 25, 37; Edmund E. Tylutki: 22; Don A. Coviello: 26; Walter Sturgeon: 30; Vic Chaplik: 38; R. H. Kurtzman, Jr.: 41; Toya Morgan: 42; remaining photos by the author.

COLOR PLATES

Kit Scates: 1, 2, 4, 5, 28; James Gailun: 3, 9, 14; Howard E. Bigelow: 6A; Emily Johnson: 8; Al Northrup: 11; George H. Harrison: 15; Ellen Trueblood: 16; Orson K. Miller, Jr.: 24; Thomas W. Martin: 30; remaining plates by the author.

DRAWINGS

All artwork by Neal MacDonald.

Index

Page entries in **boldface** *refer to illustrations.*

Personal Notes

Personal Notes

PERSONAL NOTES

Personal Notes

PERSONAL NOTES

Personal Notes

PERSONAL NOTES

Personal Notes

PERSONAL NOTES

Personal Notes

PERSONAL NOTES

Personal Notes